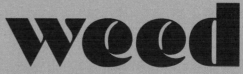

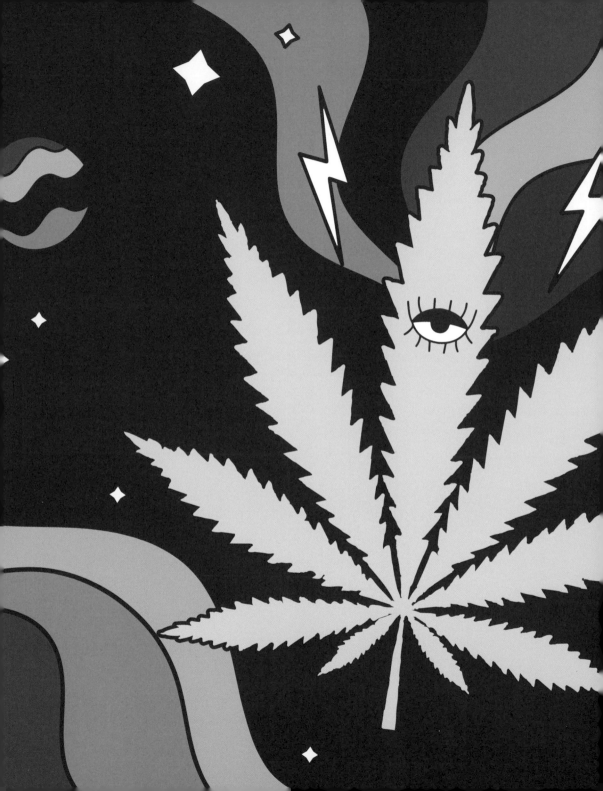

weed

Smoke It, Eat It, Grow It, Love It

Ellen Holland

EPIC INK

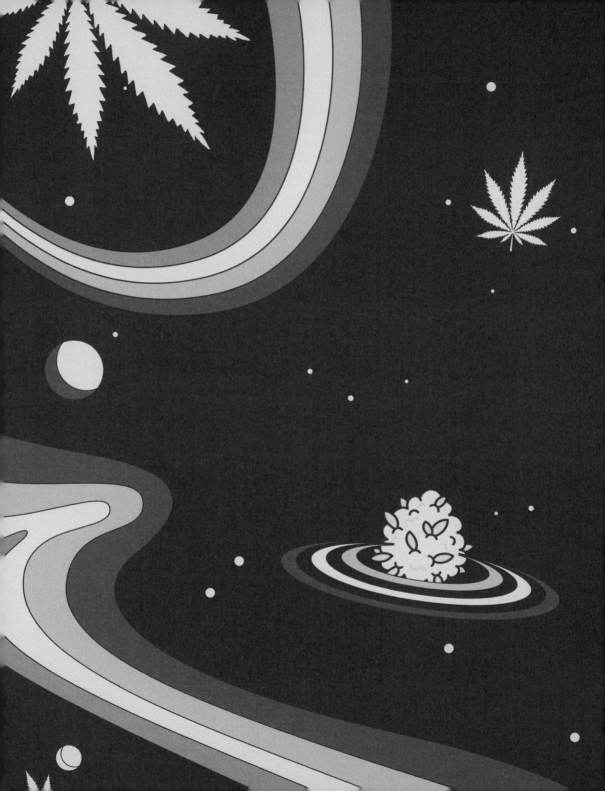

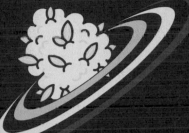

Dedicated to all those who have been
brave enough to voice their cannabis
appreciation with others.

The world is a better place for you
sharing your knowledge and your smoke.

contents

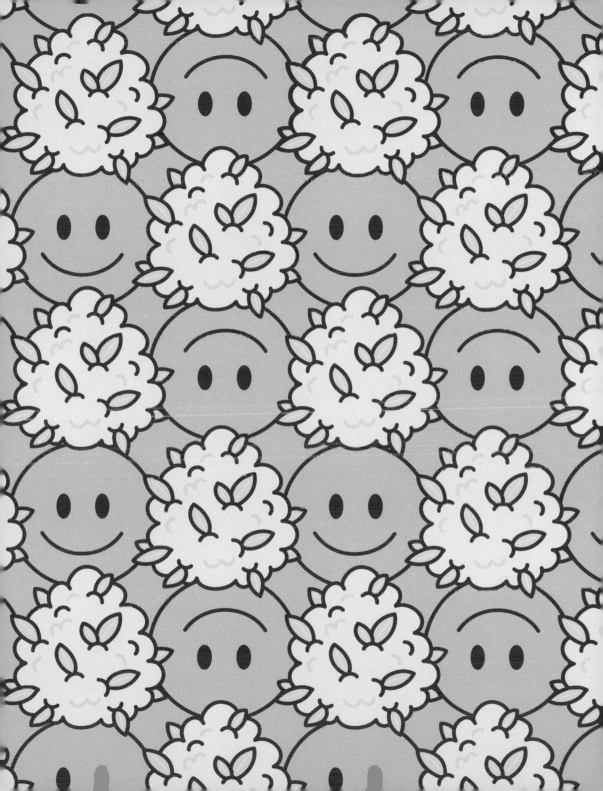

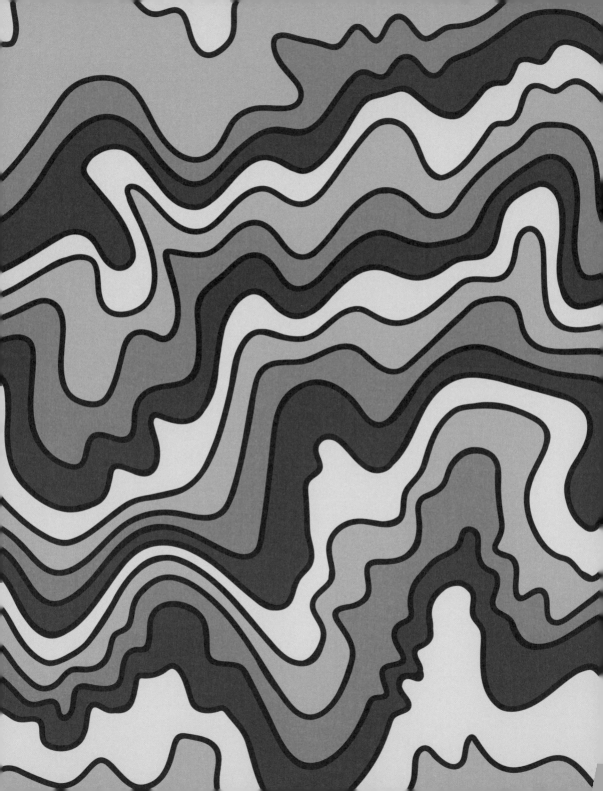

introduction

The first cannabis plant I saw in real life was on display at Oaksterdam University. America's original cannabis college had a free marijuana museum on a busy corner of downtown Oakland, California, and inside there was a grow tent with a living specimen. At the time, I didn't know anything about weed or its properties, beyond the psychoactive cannabinoid THC.

Since then, cannabis has come into its own as a product that you can acquire in storefronts across America. With this transformation also came significant headways in our understanding and appreciation of the botanical. This book takes a look at myriad ways to value this flower.

Weed is an agricultural crop with astounding biodiversity. More than half a century of breeding has resulted in thousands of different types of cannabis. This book looks at how the humble herb has risen in stature from a banned substance to a luxury product. Some tips provided by valued experts range from hosting a cannabis-tasting event to pairing pot with wine, food, and cocktails. There are also chapters on wellness practices and how cannabis can complement a path toward a healthy lifestyle.

In alignment with a healthy lifestyle, the cannabis itself should be grown in the healthiest ways possible, and several chapters provide insight into how cannabis is cultivated. California is taking unprecedented steps to preserve its heritage as the traditional breadbasket of cannabis cultivation by establishing appellations of origin that mirror those in the wine industry; the success of this program could have significant ramifications for how bud is branded and valued in the future.

With as much as we know about cannabis, there is still so much more to be discovered. My teachers and heroes lead by example in demonstrating a boundless enthusiasm toward learning more, often through personal trial and error. Through observing their intense dedication, I've developed an idea of what it means to be a cannabis expert. The most crucial components of this are learning that it's impossible to know everything and developing humility around the possibility of getting things wrong. The truth is that there are many ideal types of cannabis for each individual, which is actually a blessing because it charges you to become an expert and power your own discoveries.

This book is a guide to help protect and preserve cannabis by understanding its source, biodiversity, value, and the sheer pleasure of enjoying the perfect puff.

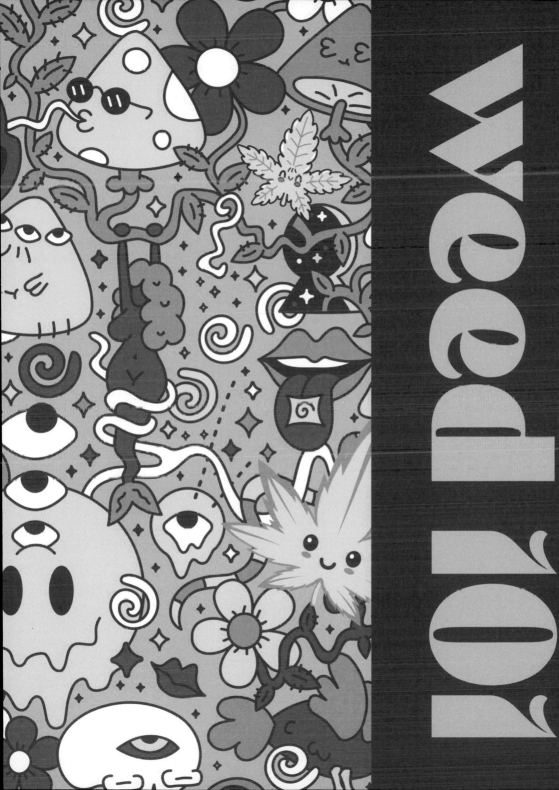

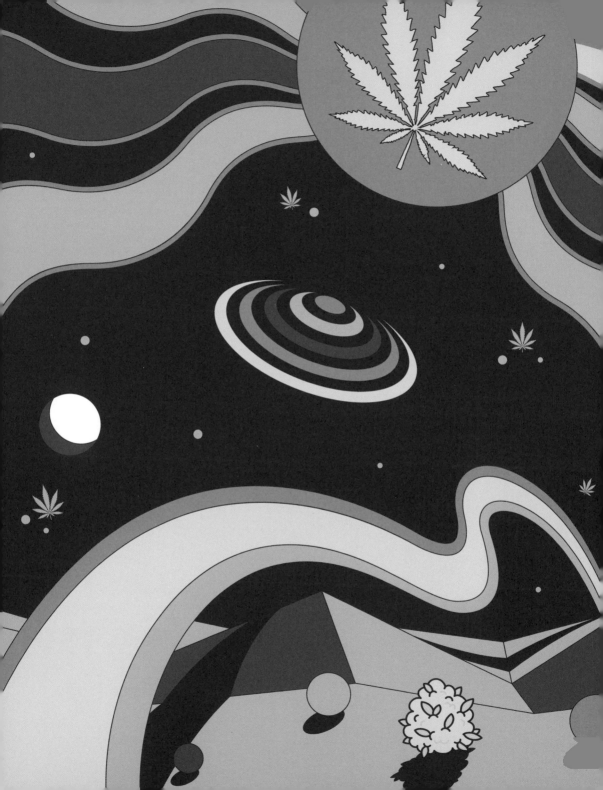

all about the aromas

The aromatic elements of the natural world, the same ones that are steam-distilled to create essential oils found in food and fragrances, play a vital role in mental and physical well-being. The essences pulled from plants are called both terpenes and terpenoids. The terms are used interchangeably, but they are different in chemical structure. Terpenes are simple hydrocarbons, an organic chemical compound composed exclusively of hydrogen and carbon atoms. Terpenoids are also essentially terpenes, but with additional chemical constituents, most often oxygen, as a result of enzyme-driven reactions within the plant.

Terpenoids and terpenes are the aromatic elements that give cannabis its depth of incredible fragrances and tastes. As the science behind how cannabis works continues to advance, studies show that not only do they make cannabis smell amazing, but they also play an essential role in understanding exactly how this plant shapes our moods.

"Terpenoids modify the cannabis experience in a variety of ways and can make it more or less sedating, extend therapeutic benefits, and potentially make cannabis safer and better overall," says Ethan Russo, one of the world's most prominent and well-respected cannabis researchers.

Tetrahydrocannabinol (THC), the primary cannabinoid that gives cannabis its psychoactive effects, has been the main focus of cannabis research since Raphael Mechoulam synthesized and isolated it in 1964. But cannabinoids such as cannabidiol (CBD) and cannabigerol (CBG) are now gaining increasing attention. The idea is that the magic of how cannabis works is in the sum of its parts, rather than by elements in isolation.

The same chemical components that have protective functioning and beneficial elements in plants can positively contribute to the defense and regulation of systems within our bodies, just like they do for the plant itself. Like antioxidants, terpenes develop in plants to prevent disease for the plant, but they can also help our bodies avoid illness.

Terpenes unleash concentrated odors that can affect our moods. One of the easiest ways to understand this phenomenon is through citrus, which is a popular aromatic in cleaning products because it acts as both a disinfectant and a deodorizer. Physiologically the smell of citrus denotes cleanliness and has a mood-elevating and immune-stimulating effect. While cultivars named after citrus fruits such as Super Lemon Haze and Lemon G contain some limonene, the terpene present in citrus fruits, it's not the dominant terpene. Super Lemon Haze contains more terpinolene than limonene, and Lemon G contains more caryophyllene. This shows how minor and major terpenes work together to give cannabis its varied effects of scents and tastes. Limes, grapefruits, lemons, and oranges are all citrus, but they also have other components that give them their distinct individual aromas and flavors.

Another terpene, pinene, is in pine needles, tea tree, and rosemary, and cannabis cultivars including Dutch Treat and Jack Herer. It's the most prevalent terpene in nature in both coniferous trees and other plants, and studies have shown it can enhance memory and cognition.

Myrcene is the most common terpene in cannabis and has a synergistic effect with THC that enhances its sedative properties. Cultivars that are heavy in myrcene (OG Kush, Granddaddy Purple) are helpful for sleep and are known to produce "couch lock," which is an effect precisely as it sounds, of being locked to the couch, unable to move. Myrcene is also in lemongrass, thyme, and mangoes.

To help unravel the complexities of marijuana's relationship to its aromas and effects, Kevin Jodrey developed a categorization system that relies on scents. Jodrey is a Humboldt, California grower, and an internationally renowned cannabis expert who previously hosted a cannabis event called the Golden Tarp Awards. This competition focused on cannabis grown through light deprivation, where growers pull tarps over outdoor crops to manipulate the natural patterns of light. The cannabis entries were grouped and judged by their aromas in the categories of fruit, floral, fuel, and earth.

"Fuel can also include things that smell chemically, floral includes things that smell spicy," Jodrey explains. "Earth means things like fresh dirt, coffee, chocolate, and wood. Fruit is all things fruit plus anything sweet."

Because any given cannabis cultivar contains an array of terpenes, these categories are more fluid than rigid. There are two major groupings in cannabis—fruit and fuel—Jodrey says. A subcategory of fruit is floral and a subcategory of fuel is earth. Using this system and understanding its subtleties, cannabis consumers can decide what type of herb is best for them, and discover what's best for them at any given moment, depending on what effects they hope to achieve. While a bright fruit cultivar is excellent in the morning, a fuel-forward selection is perfect right before bed.

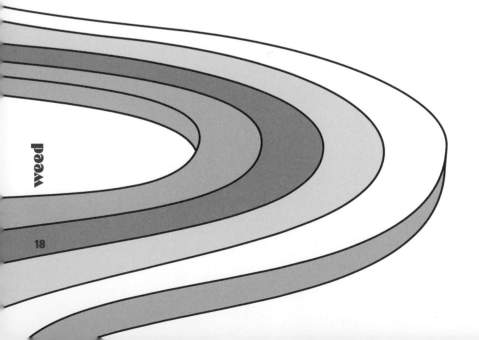

common terpenes

	Aroma
Myrcene Herbal	Musky, clove-like earthy notes
Limonene Citrus	Sweet fruit scents
Caryophyllene Peppery	Black pepper and spice
Pinene Pine	Pine needles
Linalool Floral	Floral scents
Humulene Hoppy	Woodsy earthy aromas
Terpinolene Fruity	Woodsy earth combined with citrusy pine notes
Ocimene Minty	Woodsy and sweet

Also Found In	Medical Value
Mangoes, hops, and lemongrass.	This terpene works in synergy with THC in amplifying its psychoactive effects. It's a powerful anti-inflammatory and has shown an ability to improve conditions such as osteoarthritis.
Citrus rinds and juniper.	Studies show that limonene has antimicrobial and antifungal effects. It is being studied for its ability to inhibit tumor growth and may play a role in treating cancer.
Basil, rosemary, clove, and cinnamon.	Caryophyllene activates cannabinoid receptors within peripheral tissues, the parts of the body that act as a response to a change in the environment, such as skin. It has shown progress in treating inflammation, pain, the buildup of cholesterol on artery walls (atherosclerosis), osteoporosis, and osteoarthritis.
Tea trees, rosemary, basil, and dill.	Pinene has been shown to be useful for retaining and restoring memory. Researchers are looking at pinene for treating conditions such as dementia and Alzheimer's.
Lavender, laurel, rosewood, and birch trees.	Linalool can produce sedative calming effects and reduce agitation. That means this terpene could have applications in treating conditions such as PTSD. It is also showing promise for its ability to counteract epileptic seizures.
Hops, basil, coriander, cloves, ginseng, and ginger.	Humulene has been shown to have formidable anti-inflammatory properties.
Apples, lilacs, cumin, and nutmeg.	Interest in treatments with this cannabinoid includes coronary heart disease as well as its antifungal properties.
Mangoes, orchids, mint, parsley, and basil.	Ocimene has been shown to have effective anti-inflammatory properties.

cannabinoids & the endocannabinoid system

Since it's a relatively recent scientific discovery, many traditional medical professionals are still unaware of the endocannabinoid system (ECS) and its crucial role in establishing balance within our bodies. Present in all humans as well as in animals, plants, and fungi (essentially, anything that has a cellular structure with an envelope-enclosed nucleus), the endocannabinoid system is a full-body signaling network that includes receptor sites CB1 and CB2, configured to respond to cannabinoids. These receptors are in the brain, organs, connective tissues, bones, glands, and immune cells, and the ultimate goal of their activation is so the body can maintain stability to prevent disease.

Cannabinoids function like neurotransmitters; they are involved in sending chemical messages between nerve cells, or neurons, throughout the brain, nervous, and immune systems. Interacting with the body's internal receptors are two types of cannabinoids: endocannabinoids, those produced internally, and phytocannabinoids, those found in the cannabis plant. Scientists also create synthetic cannabinoids in lab settings.

CB1

Brain
Lungs
Vascular System
Muscles
Gastrointestinal
Tract
Reproductive
Organs
Immune System
Liver
Bone Marrow
Pancreas

CB2

Spleen
Bones
Skin
Immune System
Liver
Bone Marrow
Pancreas

Human Cannabinoid Receptors

The Entourage Effect

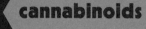

cannabinoids

terpenes

flavonoids

full-spectrum

The entourage effect explains why cannabinoids in isolation, such as Marinol, a synthetic form of THC, don't work as well as medications that incorporate other chemical elements of the plant. Turning this theory into a marketing tactic, many cannabis oils and tinctures advertise "full-spectrum" extract offerings, meaning that the product includes a range of cannabinoids and terpenes. The idea is that these products maintain the full profile of the plant and are therefore more beneficial.

common cannabinoids & effects

THC

Tetrahydrocannabinol (THC) is the most well-recognized cannabinoid because it's the one that's primarily responsible for the psychoactive effects of cannabis—the "high." Once the only measure of the quality of any given cannabis flower, this cannabinoid's brilliance over all others is only now starting to dim slightly with the rise of CBD. THC can alter the functioning of the hippocampus, the area of the brain that stores memories. THC also impacts the brain's areas associated with pleasure, concentration, movement, coordination, and time perception. It's the most prevalent of the active ingredients in cannabis. The presence of THC, more specifically 0.3 percent THC, is the arbitrary measure that defines a plant as cannabis as opposed to hemp.

CBD

Cannabidiol (CBD) is the second most-prevalent cannabinoid found in cannabis. This cannabinoid doesn't make people feel "stoned" or intoxicated and can alleviate some of the adverse effects of feeling too high. Scientists and researchers are studying CBD to treat a wide range of illnesses associated with anxiety, chronic pain, depression, and inflammation.

THCA & CBDA

The acidic precursors of what becomes THC and CBD, these cannabinoids need heat to become "active" in the traditional sense. In their raw form, these cannabinoids benefit the body by reducing inflammation and regulating the immune system.

CBN

Cannabinol (CBN) is what THC turns into as it ages. This cannabinoid has synergistic effects with THC, leading to enhanced sedative effects— meaning it's useful for treating insomnia. The easiest way to find CBN is through aged flowers.

CBG

The "mother" of all cannabinoids, cannabigerol (CBG) is the main building block for what later becomes THC and CBD. As the plant matures, enzymes break down the acidic form of CBG (CBGA) into THCA, CBDA, and CBCA (cannabichromene). The amounts of CBDA that remain after this process become CBG with heat. CBG is gaining increasing attention for its potential to treat things like inflammatory bowel disease, chronic pain, and epilepsy.

THCV

Tetrahydrocannabivarin (THCV) is a rare cannabinoid that acts as an appetite suppressant. This cannabinoid has shown an ability to treat diabetes and several other conditions, including anxiety and osteoporosis.

Memory and Depression

Cannabinoids can suppress memories, but they can also work to preserve them. The mood-altering abilities of cannabinoids show promise in treating anxiety and depression.

Appetite

Cannabinoids can increase the appetite, which is a good thing with conditions that cause nausea, although they can also decrease the desire to eat. They can be used to treat diseases like diabetes, too.

Sleep

It's common knowledge that cannabis can help with sleep. Studies suggest cannabinoids improve sleep quality, decrease disturbances, and decrease the amount of time it takes to go from fully awake to sleeping.

Stress Response

A negative response to stress stimuli can cause physical harm. The fact that cannabinoid receptors are highly assembled in the hippocampus—an area associated with memory, learning, and emotional processes— suggests that ECS signaling prevents stress and worry.

Immune Response

Cannabinoids modulate our immune system's reaction to inflammation and infection. Modulation of the endocannabinoid system interferes with cancerous cells' proliferation in two ways: either inhibiting cell signaling or inducing the death of cancerous cells.

Metabolism

The primary function of the ECS is to maintain a steady set of conditions within our bodies. In this way, the ECS is critical in regulating metabolic risk factors associated with obesity. Cannabinoids control glucose metabolism in several organs.

Endocannabinoid System Interactions

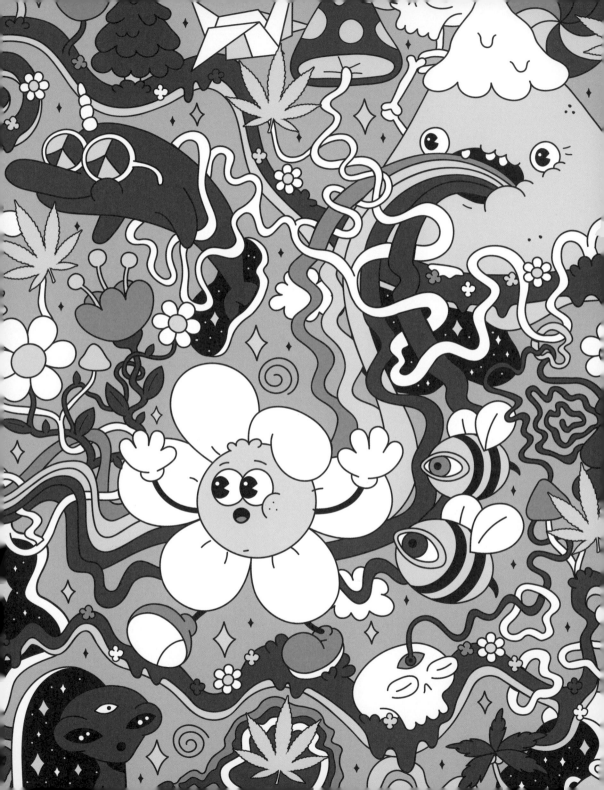

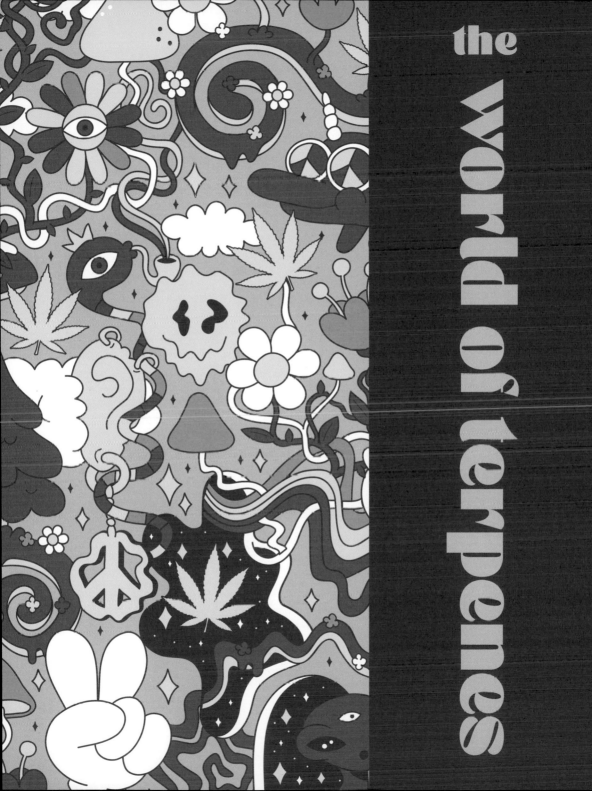

the world of terpenes

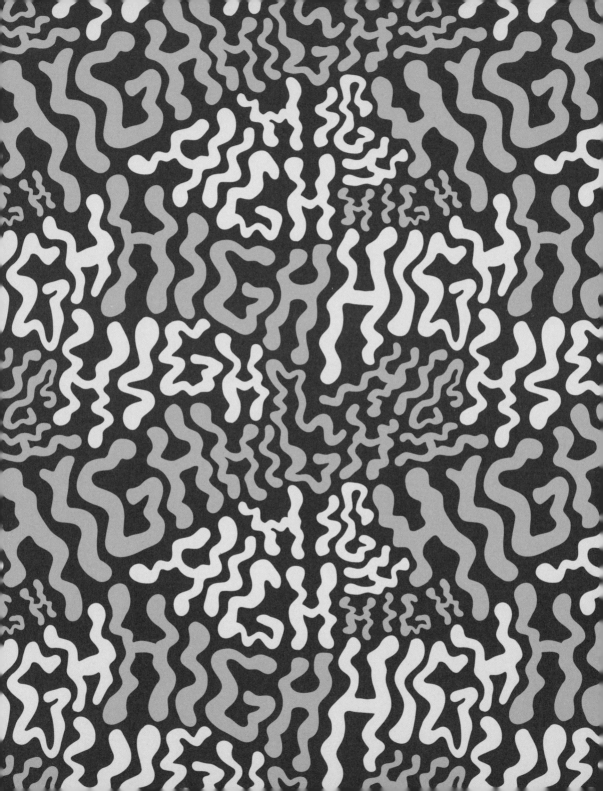

fruit salad

The spectacular rainbow of fruit flavors in cannabis encompasses everything from dark stone fruits and peaches to citrus zings and tropical tones. All deliver their own unique burst of brightness, as fruit cultivars are uplifting and unlock happy moods. Rich in terpenes like terpinolene and limonene, flowers in this category of cannabis can be authentic representations of fruits, bringing on tastes like the tartness of a blueberry or the custardy tropical cream of a mango. Fruit-forward cannabis animates the spirit and helps with a motivational push at any time of day, but they are particularly enjoyable in the morning hours. Fruity cannabis has broad appeal, delightful tastes, and energizing effects.

fruit cult classics

The cornerstone of fruit flavors in cannabis was built around the popularity of Blueberry. This cultivar's name reflects both its taste and its color, as the fresh buds take on cool blue shades that transform to a lavender hue when dried. Created by legendary breeder DJ Short, Blueberry tastes like its namesake, with sweet fruit flavors and vanilla undertones. Blueberry arrived in the 1970s and its lineage incorporates traditional cultivars known as landrace varieties (strains grown in their natural environment that have never been crossed with another type of cannabis); a Purple Thai was crossed with Highland Thai and then crossed with an Afghani.

With seeds likely smuggled across the ocean by Southern California surfers called the Brotherhood of Eternal Love, Haze (another fruit classic) and all of its progeny shaped many generations of fruit cultivars. Cannabis expert Rick Pfrommer explains that Haze, uplifting and euphoric, originated from unknown landrace cultivars via the Haze Brothers. It's a unique old-school cultivar shaped by many legends in cannabis breeding, including Dave Watson, otherwise known as Sam the Skunkman. He formed many Hazes through his partnerships with Dutch breeders and promoted two other cultivars that impacted cannabis breeding globally, Skunk #1 and California Orange.

Blueberry

Lineage	Purple Thai, Highland Thai, Afghani
Mood	Relaxed, Creative, Sleepy
RX	Depression, Insomnia, Anxiety
Taste	Vanilla, Sweet Fruit

Haze

Lineage	Unknown landrace cultivars
Mood	Focused, Creative, Euphoric
RX	Depression, Appetite, Anxiety
Taste	Sweet, Earthy

citrus scents

Smells and tastes from citrus fruits are common in cannabis. Green House created a massive hit in 2008 when it blended the Super Silver Haze with a Lemon Skunk that offered a citrusy blast of limonene. This strain, Super Lemon Haze, went on to win numerous cannabis competitions and shaped the path for many more citrus strains to follow. Classic cornerstone strains like Super Silver Haze and Super Lemon Haze eventually gave way to other citrusy aromas. One notable citrus strain was Tangie, a cross of California Orange and a Skunk created by Crockett Family Farms, which swept the sativa concentrate category of the 2015 Cannabis Cup in Denver, Colorado.

tropical terps

Cultivars with tropical flavors are also trendy fruit offerings. Crossing Ghost OG and Skunk Haze resulted in Banana Kush, which combines the fuel profile of an OG Kush with a fruity and sweet combo of Haze and Skunk. Banana flavors are big in weed. There are at least 100 cultivars with banana in the name, and new cultivars are always being created to pull from the banana flavors, which offer tastes of melon, pineapple, candy, and clove. Tropical terpene lovers can keep an eye out for Papaya crosses. This cultivar, bred by Nirvana Seeds in Holland, combines the strains Citral #13 and Ice #2 into a plant "who will really express herself once flowering begins, with a heavy onset of pistils that mature into an illuminous hypnotic orange," its breeders write. The taste of Papaya evokes fresh fruit and spices and is increasing in popularity.

candy cultivars

Fruit flavors eventually inspired cultivars that draw directly from the sugary sweetness of candy. These types of cannabis include newer selections, like Cotton Candy, Candyland, Fruity Pebbles, and Gushers; it also includes Bubble Gum, an older candy strain with an uplifting, sweet profile, which originated in Indiana in the 1970s and took on a new life when the genetics made it to Holland in the 1990s.

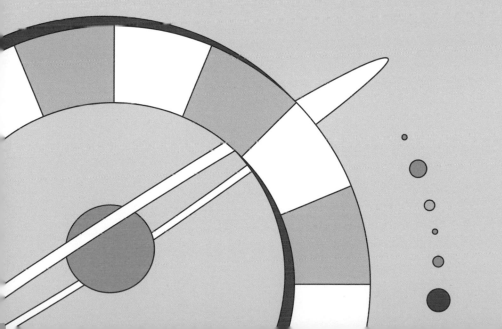

flowery aromas & tastes

Cannabis is a flower, so it's no wonder that so many types of the botanical fall into a terpene grouping on the floral side. Floral cultivars are subdivided below fruits on the flavor spectrum and share much of the same sweet structure. They can bring on bouts of inspiration and are excellent for peaceful puffs midday.

Floral cannabis cultivars are pick-me-ups that aren't quite as bright-tasting as their fruitier counterparts, but are still certainly on the uplifting side when it comes to their effects. There are all types of cannabis that branch out from blossomy scents. The warm powdery aroma of mimosa, the rich, sweet notes of lilacs, and the rose-like aromas that pull in hints of vanilla, these types of smells and tastes in cannabis cultivars are wonderful for creativity and can also be very calming.

Cultivars on the floral and earth sides do not have the pronounced aromas of those within the dominant categories of fruit and fuel, but they still offer delicious smells and tastes. Much of the floral cultivar profile originates with the work of Dutch breeders. This starts with the category's backbone, one of the main building blocks of modern-day marijuana cultivars, Skunk #1. The strain was released by Sensi Seeds in the 1980s and played a role in creating many different floral-leaning cultivars until more robust strain profiles like OG Kush and Sour Diesel drove consumer tastes toward the fuel profile in the late 1990s and early 2000s. The original version of Skunk #1, created by crossing Acapulco Gold with Colombian Gold and Afghani, resulted in many variations within several Dutch seed banks.

The Skunk cross that became iconic in representing the floral side of marijuana is Lavender, created by Soma's Sacred Seeds. Made from a mix of Super Skunk, Big Skunk Korean, and an Afghani crossed with Hawaiian, the buds on this cultivar are a violet hue, and the leaves take on such a dark shade of purple that they become almost black. Much like many cultivars with a floral composition, Lavender can be sedating, but it can also be stimulating. Its breeder, Soma, says it "produces a captivating high that circulates through every chakra." The lavender plant, which contains the same terpene found in many floral-leaning cannabis cultivars, linalool, is one of the world's oldest medicinal plants. Ancient Egyptians, Romans, and Greeks all recognized the healing powers of lavender, and clinical studies have shown that linalool has calming effects that can reduce anxiety. Linalool is also found in other plants like coriander, laurel, and birch trees. The scent of linalool is sedating and relaxing, meaning it can be a good remedy for depression. It's also an excellent sleep aid and can treat pain and modulate moods.

The terpene geraniol adds a floral sweetness with a hint of citrus and is often found in cultivars that also contain linalool. Geraniol is the primary component of rose oil and citronella oil and is also within geraniums. Like many terpenes, its smell is known to repel insects, which explains its presence in candles and sprays to keep bugs away. It's used to recreate peach, raspberry, and plum flavors and give a fresh scent to bath products.

Nerolidol is another terpene that falls in the floral category. It's also found in jasmine and has a nuanced aroma that has woodsy notes coupled with aromas of citrus, apples, and roses. This terpene is unique in that it is shown to enhance skin penetration, which could make cannabis that is applied topically more effective.

Terpinolene is the terpene responsible for the aroma and flavors in the Jack family of cannabis, derived from the Jack Herer cultivar. Named after the beloved author and hemp activist, the cultivar crafted by Sensi Seeds is a cross of multiple unknown hybrid Haze strains with a Red Skunk. Jack Herer is known for its energetic and uplifting high, making it a good companion for creative pursuits. This cultivar comes from diverse, albeit unknown, genetics and expresses complex aromas, including citrus and cedarwood, with some of the floral aspects pulled from its Skunk heritage. Terpinolene is also found in lilacs and is a beneficial terpene for those seeking relaxation or creative productivity.

Cannabis can enhance our introspective nature and has been used in rituals in many cultures. Cultivars that include an element of floral tastes and smells often push our thoughts in that direction, helping us to better assess what is going on inside ourselves and examine the world around us. Cannabis with flowery tastes and smells can offer fresh insights, but will not weigh you down, meaning they are excellent for either the morning or midday. Varietals that express floral tastes and aromas aren't heavy hitters that will be felt primarily in the body, but instead they will unlock and inspire hidden corners of the mind. Weed has a long history of contributions to inspiring great art, and cultivars within the floral profile are excellent companions for this journey.

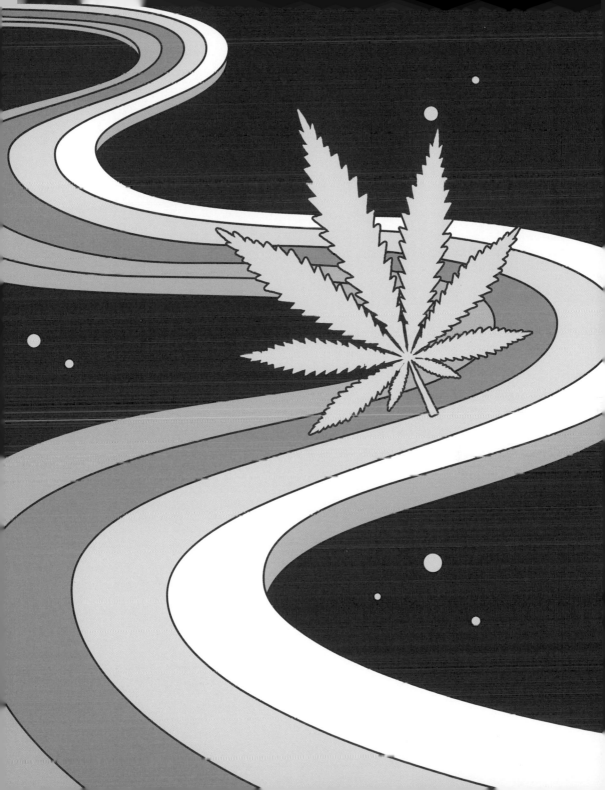

floral cult classic

Throughout the history of the cannabis plant, two places have played massive roles in developing new varieties: Amsterdam and California. Tracing the roots of cannabis cultivars back always starts at the landraces, then takes us back to one of those locations, and even more often, it's a fusion between the two.

Many selections that formed modern-day marijuana strains find their home in the earlier entries of Ed Rosenthal's *The Big Book of Buds* set, a series of books released in alignment with seed companies to announce the release of new cultivars. Among them is the legend of Skunk #1, a variety that, like the origin stories of so many cultivars, involves the work of creative minds in both California and Holland. As described by the breeder behind the Flying Dutchman seed company, in the mid-1970s, a few Dutch cultivators were growing small, average-tasting plants at home when genetics that arrived via one man changed it all. Purveyor Dave Watson's Skunk #1 was a combination of genetics from an Acapulco Gold with Colombian Gold crossed with Afghani. This became the first true hybrid in Holland's marijuana scene and wholly shaped the trajectory of things to come. Contrary to expectations that a name like "skunk" conjures, this strain has a delicate, floral taste. Its iteration released by Flying Dutchman won the first High Times Cannabis Cup held in Amsterdam in 1987.

The ultimate floral cannabis cultivar has Skunk #1 within its lineage. Lavender is a cross of two types of cannabis created with Skunk #1, Super Skunk and Big Skunk Korean, with an Afghani crossed with a Hawaiian. Another older cultivar with a floral expression is Flo. A member of DJ Short's Delta 9 Blue Collection, Flo is a cross of Purple Thai with an Afghani. It is said to have gained the name due to the plant's unique ability to produce a continual flow of buds through multiple harvests (cannabis can be regenerated to create more than one crop, but it's an uncommon practice).

Skunk #1

Lineage	Acapulco Gold, Colombian Gold, Afghani
Mood	Focused, Relaxed, Hungry
RX	Depression, Fatigue, Chronic Pain
Taste	Earthy, Sour

Lavender

Lineage	Super Skunk, Big Skunk Korean, Afghani Hawaiian
Mood	Creative, Euphoric, Sleepy
RX	Depression, Insomnia, Pain, Anxiety
Taste	Earthy, Floral

Flo

Lineage	Purple Thai, Afghani
Mood	Relaxed, Focused, Euphoric
RX	Depression, Anxiety, Pain, Nausea
Taste	Floral, Musk

chemical cuts

In the 1990s and 2000s, cannabis breeders turned up the gas. Cultivars within the fuel category are strong and have pungent notes of diesel. The thing that gives gasoline its distinctive scent, benzene, is actually a toxin in high concentrations or in long-term exposure, but its sweet odor is still appealing to many. Cannabis that falls on the fuel side mimics the odor of benzene that you'd catch at a gas station: odoriferous, almost sweet, and chemical.

Fuel-forward cultivars like OG Kush have aromas of gasoline and fresh florals. These types of cannabis also typically result in more of a body-high than a head-high; they work very well for conditions like chronic pain and are excellent for enjoying at the end of a busy day.

"Gas" is used to describe strong varieties in the same way that "loud" is, but cultivars that represent the aroma and tastes of fuel will have some sort of chemical, ammonia-like component. These are the strongest cultivars out there, powerhouses of potency that are often described as calm or relaxing. Fuel-leaning cultivars typically have large dense buds and full flavor profiles. These cultivars are incredibly pungent and chemically astringent, both in smell and smoke.

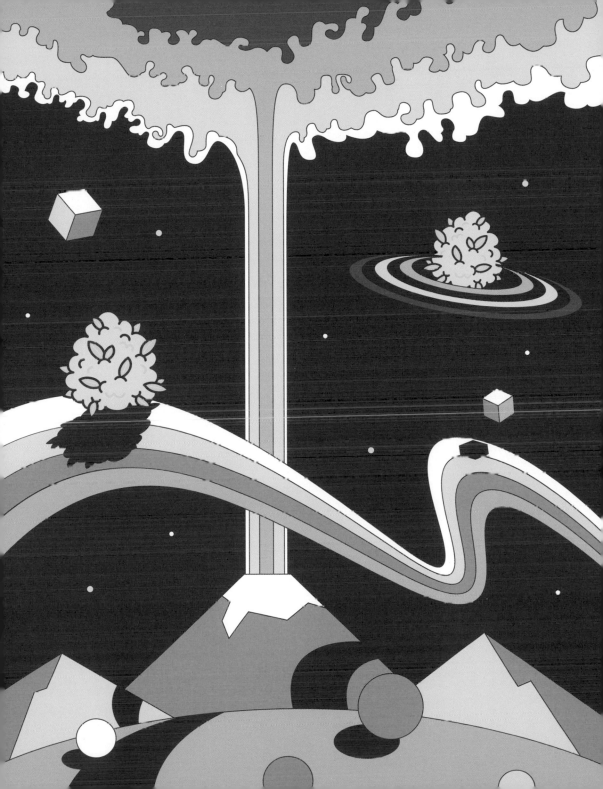

fuel cult classics

Sour Diesel stands as one of the pillars of cannabis cultivars expressing a fuel profile. It combines the scent of diesel gasoline with a burst of energy from a sour lemon tang. Like many cultivars within the fuel grouping, the exact origins of its lineage are murky. It's thought to be a cross of a Chemdog that was accidentally pollinated by a Super Skunk.

Cannabis within the fuel category of the pot palate offers rich, complex aromas. Often combining a sour citrus tang with the chemical stench of oil, these types of cannabis frequently have high THC percentages that can make them potent and sedative. Still, their citrus zing also ensures they provide just enough uplifting energy. Sour, musky, astringent, and chemical, these fuel-forward profiles take cannabis to deep, rich, dank places. Because these types of strains are so heavy, they combine well with the fruit and floral notes of citrus and candy, which pulls back a bit from some of those heady gasoline aromas and tastes.

Cultivars like OG Kush, GG4, and GSC have forever changed the pot palate with their unabashed intense aromas and tastes. While the early years of cannabis genetics had the marketplace in Amsterdam dominate the strain scene, cultivars in the fuel category showcase the best efforts on American soil and, often more specifically, the Golden State. These cultivars are pillars of cannabis genetics.

Sour Diesel

Lineage	Chemdog, Super Skunk
Mood	Focused, Creative, Euphoric
RX	Depression, Nausea, Pain
Taste	Gasoline, Citrus

OG Kush

Lineage	Chemdog, Hindu Kush
Mood	Relaxed, Euphoric, Sedated
RX	Depression, Appetite, Pain, Nausea
Taste	Gasoline, Spice

Chemdog

Lineage	Thai landrace, Nepalese landrace
Mood	Focused, Creative, Euphoric
RX	Nausea
Taste	Musk, Pine, Ammonia

from the soil

The aroma and taste of many classic types of cannabis, the landrace varietals, represent the earth's essence. With the richness of the soil, the sharp, invigorating freshness of a pine forest, the woodsy aroma of cedarwood trees, moss, bark, and roots, cannabis cultivars expressing earth are often rugged, musky, and slightly sweet. Earthy cannabis cultivars are not overwhelmingly powerful, but provide a relaxing body buzz that reduces pain, stress, and tension.

An earthy taste in cannabis reveals an ancient flavor, like worn leather or a quality miso paste. Herbal and vegetal notes are also incorporated in this taste profile, as are the roasted elements of chocolate and coffee. Earthy types of strains walk a line between sweet and savory. Earth can go from dusty aromas to more vegetal aromas, like a wet forest floor. The Kush family of strains originate from the Hindu Kush, a mountain range that stretches through Afghanistan. While OG Kush is the most familiar in the Kush family, this next-generation, fuel-forward strain originated from landraces that were more representative of the softer side of earthy tastes.

As outlined in the research article "Cannabis Taxonomy: The 'Sativa' vs. 'Indica' Debate," by Robert Clarke and Mark Merlin, Swedish botanist Carl Linnaeus came up with the scientific name *Cannabis sativa* in 1753. Considered the father of modern taxonomy, his two-part names, which often have Latin bases, convey genus first (a group marked by common characteristics), then species (a biological classification for groups capable of interbreeding). Cannabis derives from the Greek *kannabis*, and *sativa* simply means "cultivated." In 1785, European naturalist Jean-Baptiste Lamarck proposed that there were actually two species of cannabis that looked different depending on where they were grown. The plants he observed in India were shorter, with thick leaves and denser buds, and so he called them *Cannabis indica*. This designation came to describe the plants taking root in higher elevations in places like southern Asia (Nepal, China) and the Indian subcontinent (India, Afghanistan, Pakistan). The designation of *Cannabis sativa* evolved to describe plants from tropical zones close to the equator (Africa, Asia, South America). These types of cannabis were tall and lanky, with thin leaves and wispy flowers.

Cultivars that fall within the earth category of scents and tastes originate from these broad-leafed indica plants. Indica is known for producing a body buzz, while sativa is known for more cerebral effects. Varieties with earthy profiles typically have high ratios of THC, but they're not quite as strong as those cultivars that align more with the fuel profile. The earth category of cannabis is a subcategory under fuel, but earthy strains are sweeter and softer.

Cultivars with a pine taste and aroma express the terpene pinene, found in pine needles. Pinene is one of the more straightforward flavors and scents to identify in cannabis because it's so distinct. Like an invigorating walk through the forest, experiencing the olfactory benefits of pinene can be both energizing and relaxing, as well as helpful in reducing anxiety.

Chocolate and coffee are also flavors that find themselves represented in the earthy elements of marijuana. The earthiness in both involves the roasted tastes of coffee or cacao beans. In cannabis, expressing these types of flavors and tastes reveals a particular kind of natural sweetness. The warm aroma of roasted flavors adds complexity to cultivars that incorporate chocolate or coffee tastes and smells.

Cacao produces the cannabinoid anandamide, which is the same one that our bodies create internally to activate feelings of bliss. Anandamide binds to the same receptors in the brain as THC, explaining why many people say eating chocolate or smoking marijuana brings them joy. Combining the mood-enhancing properties of eating chocolate with those from smoking cultivars that evoke those same scents, tastes, and feelings is an excellent method for adding to the overall sensory experience of enjoying this flower.

Interestingly, coffee also targets our endocannabinoid systems. Coffee decreases the effects of cannabis, which helps to unpack why it can be used as a tool to sober up those who may be feeling the adverse effects of being too high. Earthy cannabis cultivars evoke rustic elements that feel familiar. Cannabis described as earthy will have the aroma and flavors of soil, minerals, and vegetation and likely has close roots to landrace lineage. These types of cannabis are perfect for promoting peaceful moments of calm and are an excellent option for those looking to unwind the mind and body.

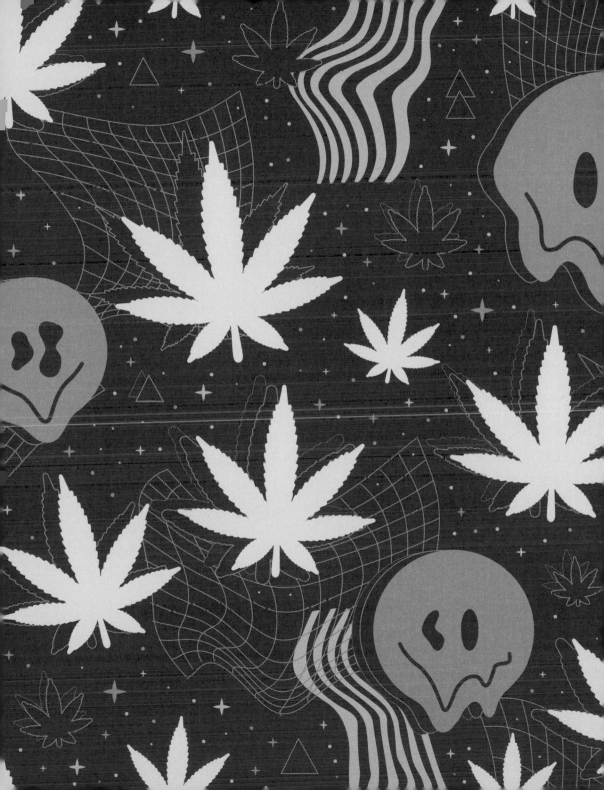

earth cult classics

When it comes to earthy cannabis, the cultivars don't stray far from marijuana's beginnings. Landrace cannabis forms the backbone of all modern-day cultivars, but with cannabis that's earthy, the essential elements don't differentiate much from the past's classic tastes and aromas. Incorporating flavors that range from fresh earth and minerals to woody and pine scents, earth is an element of weed's flavor and scent profile with a wide range. While aspects of earthy cannabis cultivars can be stimulating, these strains are often calming and optimal for alleviating mental stress or physical pain.

Many cannabis cultivars pick up the flavors of the classic Kush varietals that originate from the Hindu Kush mountains on the earthy end of the spectrum. Unlike those strains that lead to more chemical, gassy aromas and tastes, earthy strains stay on the softer, sweeter side.

Earth is an essence that runs through many different types of cannabis. More subtle than fruit or fuel, earth is similar to floral in offering softer tastes. Smells of the woods present in cannabis terpenes are also within pine, cedar, eucalyptus, bay laurel, oak, juniper, and tea trees. Spices and herbs like nutmeg, clove, pepper, basil, and rosemary also have terpenes found in cannabis that have an earthy side. Whether they are woodsy or rich notes of soil, these types of cannabis can be savory or sweet, but they generally reveal ganja's more relaxing side.

Hindu Kush

Lineage	Afghani landrace
Mood	Relaxed, Sleepy, Euphoric
RX	Nausea
Taste	Spice, Pine, Sandalwood

Bubba Kush

Lineage	OG Kush, Northern Lights
Mood	Relaxed, Sleepy, Euphoric
RX	Depression, Anxiety, Pain, Insomnia
Taste	Chocolate, Coffee, Spice

Gelato

Lineage	Sunset Sherbert, Thin Mint Girl Scout Cookies
Mood	Relaxed, Creative, Euphoric
RX	Nausea, Depression, Anxiety, Pain
Taste	Earthy, Berries, Cake

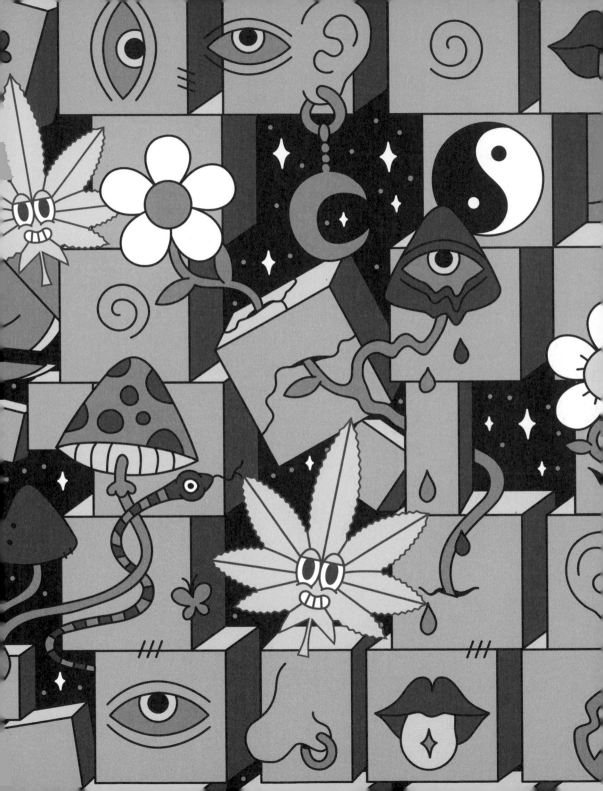

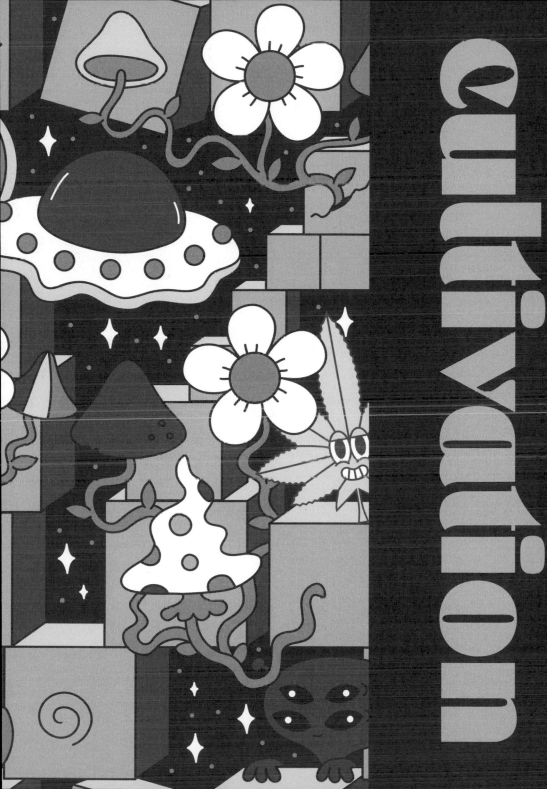

cultivation

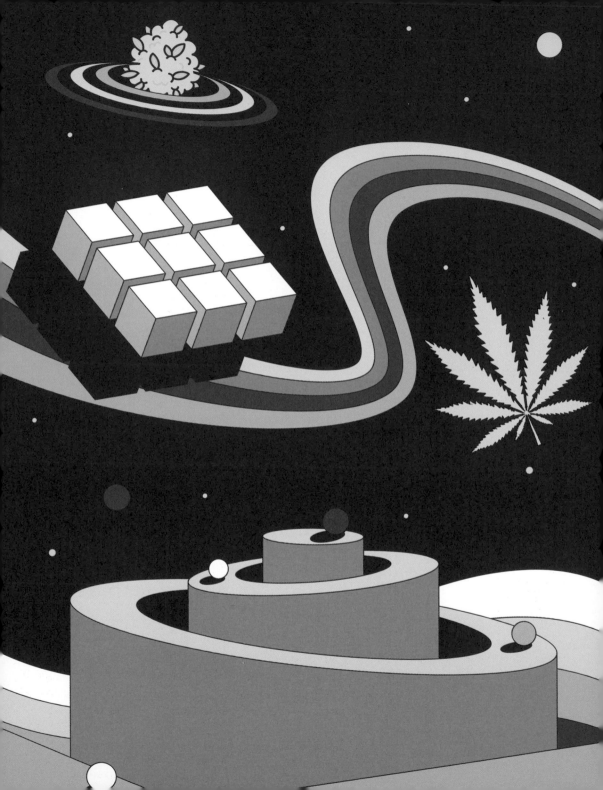

outdoor herb

Growing the plant that produces the world's most favored flowers is only considered complex because prohibition has made it so. With the right growing conditions, an open, sunny environment, well-drained soil, adequate ventilation, and sufficient nutrients and water, growing marijuana is relatively easy. However, its illegality made it necessary to take the herb out of the sun and hide it indoors. Indoors, the annual plant takes on a whole new speed of growth, as cultivators manipulate the lighting to bring the plants into flowering sooner. Unlike crops such as corn that have been commodified down to only a few types, cannabis has been lovingly formed into a prismatic array of cultivars by blending male and female plants' best attributes. The most advanced cannabis cultivators are breeders who create new flavors for an ever-hungry public and, as the channels of cannabis commerce continue to gain legitimacy and transparency, crops grown under the sun are gaining a following as passionate and enthusiastic as those who prize indoor flowers.

growing basics

Grown outdoors, cannabis is an annual crop cultivated within the growing season from spring through fall. Cannabis is dioecious, meaning the plants naturally reproduce through wind carrying pollen from the male plants to flowers on female plants. Breeders replicate this action by brushing pollen directly onto female flowers and growing out enough generations of the plant that its seeds become a stabilized, re-creatable expression.

Anyone other than a breeder sexes their plants early, separating the males from the females to ensure the female plants do not become pollinated and spend energy on producing seeds rather than buds.

plant life cycle

Cannabis seeds for outdoor grows are sown in the spring, between February and April, and germinate within a week. The fascinating part about cannabis seeds is they keep, which means that not only can they be collected to preserve genetic information, they can be grown out any number of years later.

Cannabis has two distinct stages of growth that respond to the light cycle. During the first stage, the plant responds to the increasing light by producing vegetative growth—leaves and branches. During the second stage, the shorter autumn days cause the female plant to flower. The magic number for most cultivars to flower is 12:12; in other words, it will flower when a day has twelve hours of light and twelve hours of uninterrupted darkness. Once a plant begins to flower, it will take about seven to nine weeks to finish. Indoors, the light schedules can be manipulated to reduce the time a plant spends in vegetative growth to make it flower sooner. Indoor growers are also not limited to one crop per year.

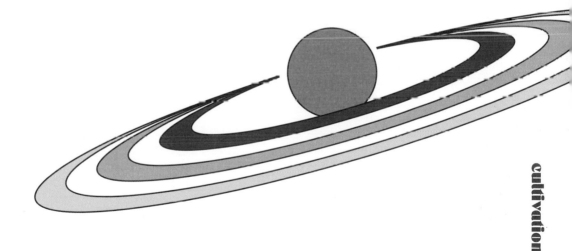

cultivation

The Cannabis Taxonomy Debate

The main thing to consider about cannabis's ecological evolution is how humanity shaped the plant to grow according to our desires by breeding it for the features we were seeking. All cannabis is under one species classification, *Cannabis sativa*, and the most fundamental split from this comes with division at two subspecies: hemp and drug. In other words, rope and dope. Hemp and cannabis are the same species, but one has been grown for fiber and the other for the mind-altering components present in its flowers' resin. What makes a plant hemp as opposed to cannabis is the presence of THC, in a calculation set in the United States at 0.3 percent.

Other taxonomy further splits the plant to include three species: *Cannabis sativa*, *Cannabis indica*, and *Cannabis ruderalis*. While it's all cannabis, plants are defined by the structure of their growth and leaves to determine their effects. Tall plants with thin leaves, long flowering times, and uplifting highs are sativas, and short, squat plants with broad leaves, shorter flowering times, and powerful sedative effects are indicas.

Some plants fall under the uncommon designation of ruderalis. These are small plants that possess the ability to flower based on the plant's maturity rather than the cycle of light; this is known as "auto-flowering."

The classifications of different types of cannabis are evolving away from traditional designations of indica and sativa as our understanding of the properties of cannabis continues to grow. While there are still landrace varietals (cannabis that dates back to before the 1960s that has not been hybridized, and so imparts the unique tastes of place), most types of cannabis have been heavily bred and blended so that they all essentially became hybrids rather than true indicas or sativas. In this way, cannabis classifications are moving away from observable physical traits like height and leaf structure and toward chemotypes (a way to classify cannabis based on its chemical constituents like cannabinoids and terpenes).

Cannabis
Indica

Cannabis
Sativa

Cannabis
Ruderalis

cultivation

59

indoor cannabis

Filled with rows and rows of fragrant living plants, indoor cannabis grows are special places. Within this land of light and darkness, the world's natural elements are recreated, manipulated, and optimized to produce the best possible result. By working with light, a plant that was once an annual crop becomes something that can now be harvested year-round. Indoor cannabis provides a consistency that growing outside cannot. With more precise control over the outcome, indoor growing can produce beautiful flowers with astounding THC percentages and incredible tastes.

In terms of lighting, growers can choose from fluorescents, high-intensity discharge (HID) lights and LEDs. HID lights include metal halide bulbs and high-pressure sodium (HPS) lights. Back in the day, most growers were still just hanging bulbs from their ceilings, then improvements like ballasts and reflective hoods came along to better regulate and increase light flow. In 2010, the Holland-based company Gavita invented the double-ended HPS light, which included a more stable ballast and put the electricity output to a much more efficient use. Then came controllers, which made the indoor cannabis grow-light setups even more precise.

With the combination of better lights and the ability to move plants placed on shelves with rollers around the space, the growing canopy can take up all of the available space and the flowers can make more efficient use of the light.

the perfect blend

Indoor grow setups come in varying scales that range from giant industrial warehouse spaces to closet grows. Many home growers still use grow tents or grow boxes (which come complete with other elements such as lights and fans) to establish a contained space for growing indoors due to space constraints.

The key to growing cannabis is the recurring cycle of uninterrupted periods of dark and light. To flower, most cultivars require a lighting regime of twelve hours on followed by twelve hours off. Outdoors, that stage of light happens as the days grow shorter in the fall, but indoors, growers choose when to bring the plant into flower by timing their lights.

Plants start as seedlings and take off during the vegetative growth stage when the roots and foliage develop. In this vegetative period, indoor plants typically receive anywhere from eighteen to twenty hours of light. Then, there are different styles of growth. Those looking for larger, bushier plants can let this vegetative period extend for a month or two. Others who grow within the "Sea of Green" style will limit the vegetative stage to a shorter amount of time because they are interested in cultivating a larger number of smaller plants closer together.

cultivation

flower power

The power and potency of pot is in the cannabis flower. When the lights are switched to 12:12, the plants devote all their energy toward flower production. Most cultivars will stay in the flowering period for seven to nine weeks, but sativas, taller plants with less chlorophyll than indicas, can take longer for the buds to properly ripen.

During the first week of flowering, the plant will work double-time to stretch and form all the buds. As flowering progresses, the buds will start to create white pistils that look like wispy hairs within the flowers. When the stretching ends, the buds will really begin to develop, becoming more prominent and fatter. They will also become a lot stickier as trichomes develop. The flowers of plants that are still in growth give off an intense perfume that goes beyond the flower's aroma once they have been dried and cured.

The trichomes reveal the information about whether or not a plant is ready to harvest, as they show the flower's ripeness. To determine this, growers use a magnifying loupe to closely examine the buds. There are different methodologies behind assessing the ripeness of cannabis plants. Still, most growers generally accept that cloudiness within the trichome heads, when they turn milky white and a few turn amber, determines the best time to harvest a plant at peak ripeness.

the indoor domination

Cannabis came indoors when it became an illegal substance; by controlling and amplifying aspects of the natural world, breeders worked with the botanical to bring out specific characteristics that they were looking for. This often only meant high THC profiles. After all, THC was not only the thing that consumers were looking for, but there also wasn't as much understanding about how terpenes in synergy with cannabinoids play a role in producing a high.

Today, the dialogue between whether growing indoors or growing outdoors is superior is getting even more nuanced as indoor growers work to improve their functioning in terms of lighting, cooling, and dehumidifying, and being better stewards of the environment. Greenhouses also continue to grow in popularity, as do light-deprivation techniques, which limits the plants' exposure to sunlight, forcing them into flowering sooner. Light deprivation integrates methods of both indoor and outdoor growing, and high-end setups will work with natural light from the sun and supplemental lighting.

regenerative agriculture

The main concept of regenerative agriculture is improving the quality of the land and, in turn, resisting the climate crisis by restoring soil diversity and reducing carbon output. When it comes to cannabis, these growing practices are being adopted by a group of community-minded farmers with an interconnected web to share ideas, trade genetics, and swap stories.

Regenerative Cannabis Farming is an organization made up of a group of volunteers who "believe regenerative land use is the key to restoring our environment, bolstering our communities, and providing holistic medicine to patients." The organization is focused on bringing awareness to the cannabis community about regenerative farming techniques. It also recognizes small farms for their commitment to the environment and the community and establishes high expectations for regenerative practices, which they believe are necessary for shifting the paradigm of resource-intensive land use.

Beyond the beneficial effects that regenerative farming has for the environment, those who grow and smoke cannabis that has been produced in a regenerative manner will tell you it also tastes the best. This type of herb takes advantage of the full spectrum of natural light and organic inputs to blossom to its fullest expression. Rich in terpenes that deliver a diverse assortment of smells and tastes, regenerative farming practices often improve flavor and bud structure, resulting in densely packed buds expressing their terroir's rich tastes (terroir is a French word that describes a sense of place).

Regenerative farming practices involve things such as cover crops, companion plants, composting, and crop rotation. These types of cannabis farms see themselves as shepherds of the earth, and they often understand cannabis as more of a sacred plant, with the powers to impart its ancient wisdom and transform our minds as well as the land where it grows.

landrace strains and their origins

Landraces are the oldest, purest strains of cannabis and the foundational building blocks of marijuana. Cannabis grown on a larger scale is often more of a commodity crop, with growers sticking to a few types of cultivars. This strategy makes good business sense, particularly in legal marketplaces where each variety must be tested at cost. But those lucky growers that do have a bit of room and the funds to play with growing new varieties display the palpable excitement of experimentation combined with curiosity. Marijuana is a fun plant to grow, and its variance means it's a puzzle that can be solved via millions of combinations. Still, with all of this diversity, sometimes it's nice to go back to the classics and remember where marijuana came from.

Landrace cannabis isn't really a cultivar because it hasn't been cultivated. This is the cannabis that has adapted to the area where it originates. These types of cannabis have not been bred to express specific characteristics, but rather to exhibit traits that allow them to thrive within the geographical region where they are

Hindu Kush
Afghanistan

Thai
Thailand

Jamaican Lion
Jamaica

Acapulco Gold
Mexico

Durban Poison
South Africa

Colombian Gold
Colombia

Panama Red
Panama

based. Landrace strains exist from before plant breeding brought out the artificial selection of characteristics; this type of cannabis has not been manipulated by human efforts.

The relationship forged between cannabis and humanity began more than 10,000 years ago. Since then, many cultures have used cannabis in different forms for different purposes and have carried the seeds to every corner of the earth. Landrace varietals exhibit the sort of vigor one would come to expect from a plant that has adapted and evolved to survive on its own. These strains were rediscovered by the experimental counterculture of the 1960s and 70s, when people preserved the seeds and worked to begin the first wave of cannabis breeding. Landrace cannabis originating from areas like Mexico, Colombia, southeast Asia, Africa, and the Hindu Kush hippie trail (a pot pilgrimage undertaken from the 1950s through the '70s) were adapted by breeders interested in creating quick-growing plants suitable for indoor environments; these plants adapted to the locations in which they were grown. Then in the 1960s, breeders in California and Holland crossbred cannabis, resulting in one of the most biodiverse plants the world over, a genetic journey that has since diversified a dozen varieties into thousands. Classic landrace strains include Jamaican Lion, Colombian Gold, Panama Red, Hindu Kush, Thai, Durban Poison, and Acapulco Gold.

Cannabis landraces represent the most venerable form of marijuana. They are the purest forms of the original representations of the plant that can be found. Rare, and at risk of extinction, these genetics are sought after by people looking to understand marijuana's past and preserve its legacy for the future.

cultivation

From Wine to Weed

California already has appellations in place within its wine industry. It's a tiered system with small, specialized zones, larger regions, and a statewide designation to show where the grapes have been grown. In wine, appellations are defined either by political boundaries, such as counties, or federally recognized growing regions called American Viticultural Areas. For example, strict rules determine that champagne only comes from Champagne, France; it's sparkling wine otherwise. France has hundreds of appellations, mostly for wine, but also for cheese, lavender, and honey.

The Californian program is less strict than the one set up in France, and cannabis is set to follow a similar path to the California program for wine through the Cannabis Appellations Program, which is being coordinated through the California Department of Food and Agriculture (CDFA). As growing cannabis becomes more transparent in legal marketplaces, the authenticity of how and where it developed will determine the value placed upon the end product. Like the high price point that winemakers in Napa Valley can get for a cabernet, the idea is that cannabis grown in a specific region could command a premium price.

branded bud

By bringing more awareness about where and how cannabis is grown, cultivators are hopeful the California cannabis appellations will allow them to market their crops in a way that's never been done before. While connoisseurs are more than willing to pay a premium for herb of the highest quality, its previously illegal nature makes it hard for consumers to trust what they are receiving. The California cannabis appellations program's standards will allow for industry-wide measures to make consumers more confident that what they see is what they get. It ensures that a product is grown where and how it indicates on its label or through its advertising. Small farmers can capitalize on the value that smokers place on unique and local cultivars. The system is designed to allow for a market where small farmers can survive and push back against the concept of cannabis as a commodity product.

Within the conversation about cannabis appellations is the idea of recognizing the heritage of cannabis within the state and preserving the legacy of small farmers and the types of specialty boutique weed that they produce. Appellations define the relationship between the land, the climate, and the final product and pull the plant ever forward as a desired luxury product.

cultivation

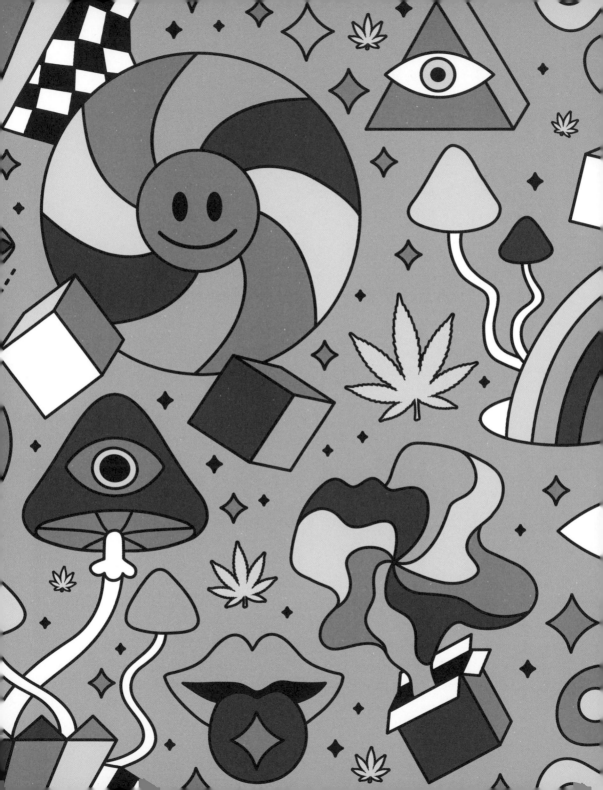

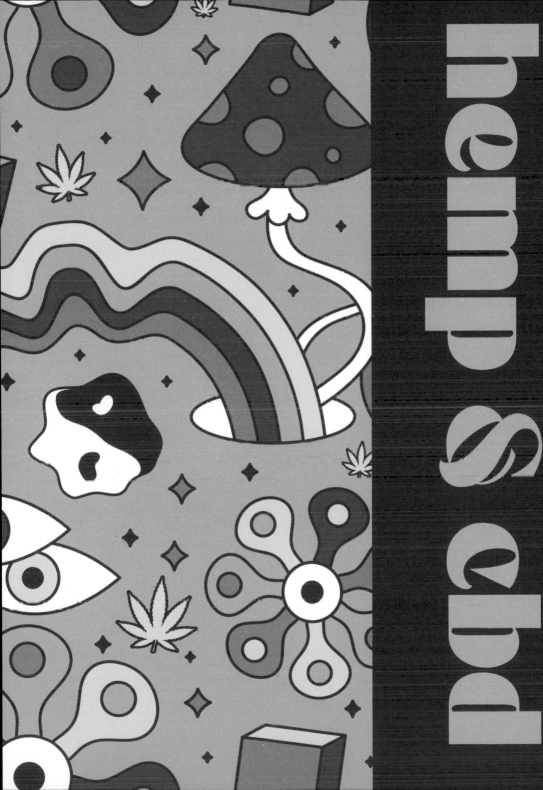

Hemp and cannabis are the same species. The difference between these plants is that they've been bred to express distinct attributes. The threshold between what defines a plant as hemp or cannabis lies in an arbitrary distinction of how much THC they contain. In the US, plants with any more than 0.3 percent THC are cannabis, while plants with less than 0.3 percent THC are hemp.

Even though CBD was being studied as a medicine, the bread basket of American cannabis genetics, California, was mostly focused on cultivars expressing a high THC profile. A group of journalists wanted to change that. In 2009, Project CBD, a nonprofit organization dedicated to promoting and publicizing information about CBD's medical applications, was founded. Headed by co-founder and director Martin Lee, a well-respected cannabis expert and the author of *Smoke Signals: A Social History of Marijuana—Medical, Recreational and Scientific*, the group felt that the reintroduction of CBD genetics into the grass-roots supply was an important moment in cannabis, and this has proven to be true. Back in 2009, it was rare to see a cannabis cultivar with CBD, but since then, growers have been breeding CBD-rich strains back into the gene pool and the market has exploded with several different elite medicinal varietals.

Because cannabis and hemp are the same except for how much THC they contain, CBD can be obtained from either source, but the hemp path has proven more accessible than the cannabis path. With the passage of the 2018 Farm Bill, hemp became legalized in the US, and many people across the country opted to navigate through the new legalized system to grow hemp.

CBD also continued to make advances in the UK, which officially declared the cannabinoid a medicine in October of 2016. The complexities and vagueness of the laws governing CBD in the UK have given rise to a profitable, competitive, and mostly unregulated system.

In June 2018, the Food and Drug Administration (FDA) approved GW Pharmaceuticals' Epidiolex® as a CBD-based treatment for two severe pediatric seizure disorders, Lennox-Gastaut syndrome and Dravet syndrome. This marked a significant turning point in terms of marijuana's applications as a pharmaceutical medication.

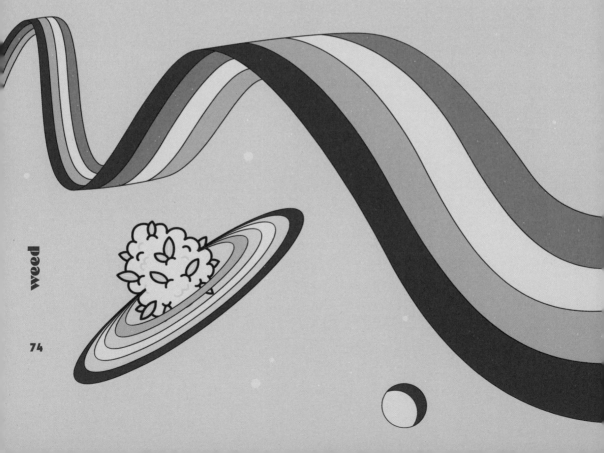

hemp in history

It's very likely that humans first discovered hemp while hunting for food sources and found the seeds to be worthwhile. Searching for other uses for the plant, the oil from hemp seeds was extracted and used in things like cooking. The fiber from the stalk was used to create objects like ropes and hemp cloth. Hemp followed this path as an excellent source for fiber and food and cannabis (the same plant now known under a different name), then embarked on a journey that focused on developing it for female flowers. More specifically, developing the psychoactive properties of its THC-laden female flowers.

The history of hemp also has deep roots in the history of America. It was one of the first crops cultivated by early colonial settlers, introduced in New England in 1629. Used for making paper and clothing, it was so valued as a cash crop in the early days of America that, in 1762, Jamestown, Virginia, imposed penalties on those who did not produce it. Even George Washington grew hemp. In diary entries from 1765, he writes about separating the male from the female hemp and pulling the seed for hemp.

When hemp's dominance as a crop to produce fibers for clothing was changed by the cotton gin's invention, the plant's focus started to shift to medicine. Hemp entered the *United States Pharmacopeia*, a drug reference manual, in 1851, and was then recommended for a wide variety of disorders.

In 1937, the Marihuana Tax Act effectively put an end to the production of cannabis and hemp in America. As they were still lumped together as one plant, the Marihuana Tax Act made growing cannabis impossible by way of imposing prohibitive costs. The Tax Act required cannabis farmers to register with the government to raise the crop. The going price of a pound of cannabis in 1937 was thirty-eight cents, the tax imposed upon its transfer for those who were legally registered was one dollar per ounce. For those who transferred it illegally, the tax was one hundred dollars an ounce. During World War II, hemp was so valuable for the war effort that the government encouraged Americans to grow the crop.

In 1970, marijuana and hemp were placed in the Controlled Substances Act (CSA) as a Schedule I substance, meaning one with no medical value. Hemp seeds and fiber were still allowed but were no longer able to be grown in the US. It wasn't until 2014 that growers in Kentucky, Vermont, and Colorado started growing hemp again on American soil, through the provisions of research programs allowed through the 2014 Farm Bill. The later 2018 Farm Bill opened the hemp market nationwide by legalizing the crop under the definition that it has less than 0.3 percent THC. This action removed hemp from the CSA, taking it out of the DEA's enforcement and placing it under the regulation of the Department of Agriculture, which oversees the nation's crop and food products.

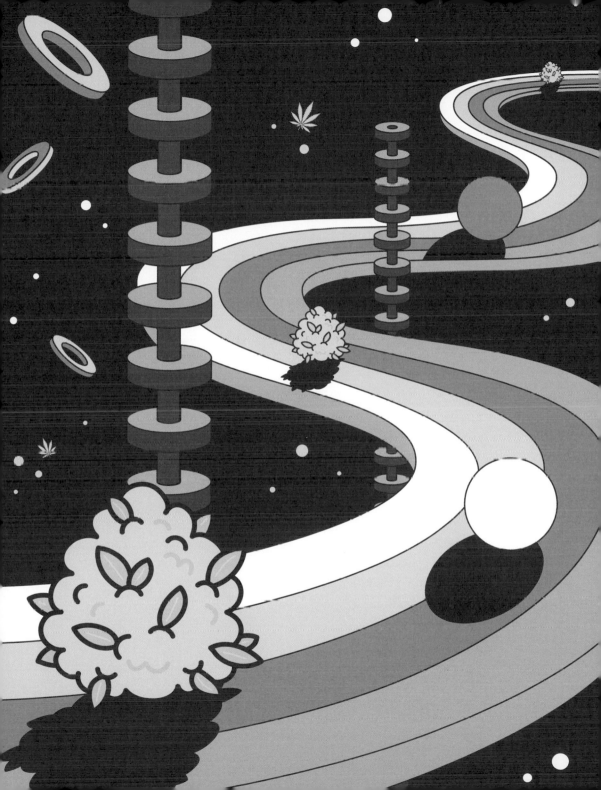

cbd as a medicine

CBD is not intoxicating, but it's a mistake to say it's non-psychoactive, because the cannabinoid does have the ability to alter our moods. Scientific research on the cannabinoid shows promise in treating things like anxiety and depression, along with things like chronic pain and inflammation. CBD also has neuroprotective qualities and, in this way, is being looked at as a potential treatment for conditions such as Alzheimer's, Parkinson's disease, dementia, epilepsy, and traumatic brain injuries.

One interesting particular application of CBD has to do with its ability to enhance the growth and strength of bones. Bone density can be affected by conditions such as osteoporosis, where bones become more porous and fragile. Studies have shown that CBD can play a positive role in restoring and preserving bone mass.

Another medical application where CBD shows promise is in conditions involving the gut, such as colitis, Crohn's disease, and irritable bowel syndrome (IBS). Cannabinoid receptors exist within the stomach's nerves, and the endocannabinoid system plays essential roles in regulating the two main functions of the gut, the digestion of food, and immune cell response to viruses and bacteria.

CBD is also being studied for its anti-cancer properties. Cannabinoids have been shown to help fight cancer in several ways, including stopping tumor growth by triggering cell death and preventing new growth, as well as preventing cancer cells from infecting other areas of the body.

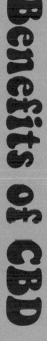

BRAIN

Antipsychotic

Antidepressant

Anti-anxiety

Antioxidant

Neuroprotective

EYES

Vasorelaxant
for glaucoma

HEART

Prevents plaque
buildup in
arteries

Anti-
inflammatory

Anti-ischemic

STOMACH

Anti-emetic

Appetite control

INTESTINES

Anti-prokinetic

HAND

Analgesic for
rheumatoid ar-
thritis

LEG

Stimulating new
bone growth

Strengthening
bones affected
by osteoporosis

Benefits of CBD

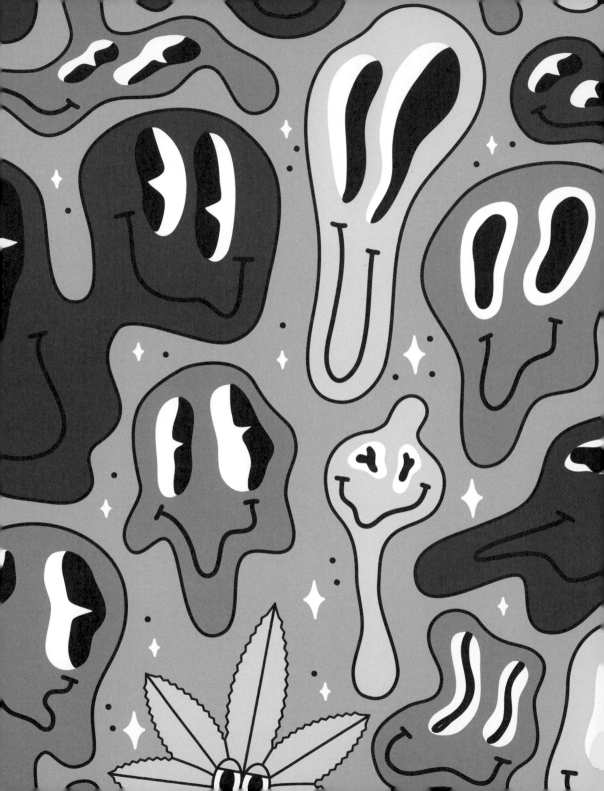

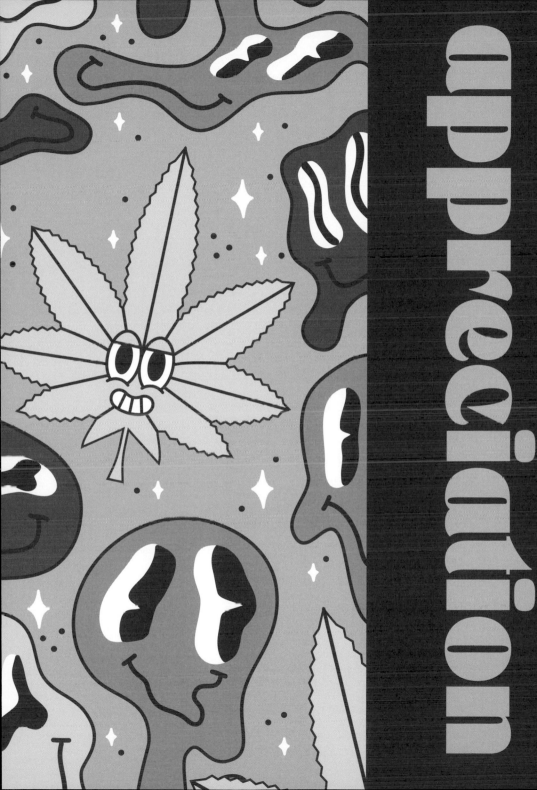

appreciation

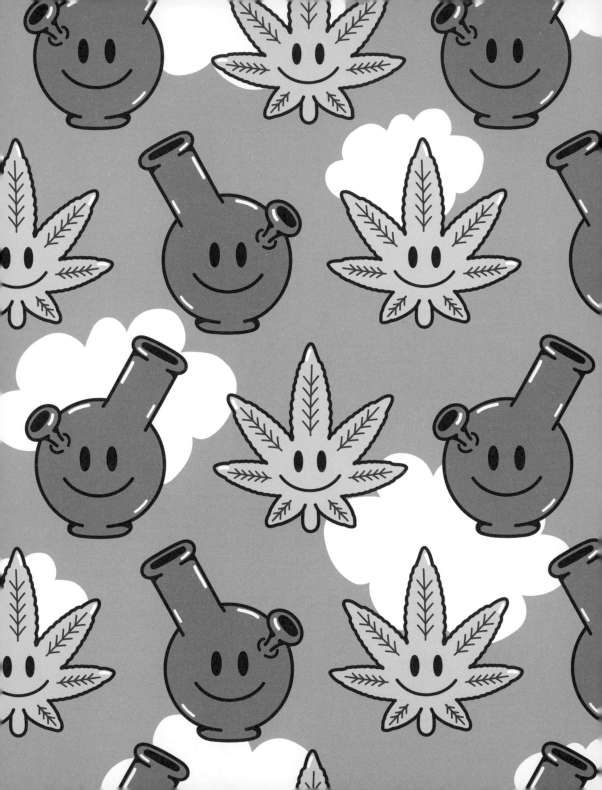

the sensory pleasures of tasting cannabis

Hosting a cannabis tasting is a great way to explore the full expression of the flower. Whether it's a blind or open tasting, sampling different types or cultivar groupings is an excellent method for getting further acquainted with the botanical's vast diversity.

For a private taste test at home, decide what type of tasting you're going to hold. Perhaps find five different cultivators who have grown the same cultivar and conduct a blind tasting to uncover the depth present in a single type of cannabis. Or look at it like a flight and get to know a single producer by tasting a selection of the cultivars they grow.

Tasting cannabis with unknown origins (that is, a blind tasting) is an experimentation with the sensory elements of cannabis that allows tasters to further grasp the inexhaustible richness and complexity the plant offers. Caitlin Podiak, a Mendocino-based outdoor cannabis expert behind the website Certified Dank, recommends participants be ready to discuss all the intricacies with the focused attention and reverence that come with enjoying any high-end product, whether the tasting is blind or open.

"Everything that goes into the cultivation of a cannabis flower matters: genetic lineage, how it's grown, where it's grown, the attitude and approach of the farmer, the care with which the plant is handled, etc.," Podiak says. "There's an enormous difference

appreciation

83

between flowers cultivated in ideal or less than ideal conditions, and I believe that most people are capable of appreciating that distinction when they have the opportunity to compare a variety of samples."

To begin, make sure everyone has paper and a pen for taking notes. At Certified Dank tastings, Podiak creates a template to outline the necessary steps and clear categories to assess the cannabis by its aroma, flavor, and effect. The basic steps? Smell the flowers, hit the joint without lighting it (something known as a dry hit), use a hemp wick to light the buds, then, finally, ask yourself what do you taste? How do you feel?

Look for color, size, density, and moisture levels. Is the cannabis solid and sticky, or more airy and dry? This is the time to notice how the buds have been trimmed and, if available, to bring out a microscope and get a close-up look at the resinous part of the plant that holds most of its properties, the trichome heads.

Unless the plan is for a rigorous blind tasting, participants can share their observations. The reasoning behind a decision to keep the tasting more tight-lipped comes into play when rating or judging cannabis on a professional scale; this is done to not unduly influence others.

Once the buds have been ground, it's time to smell them to gather more information about the flower. Does the cultivar express fuel or earth, or does it lean on the spectrum's fruity and floral end? Simply smelling cannabis is one of the best indicators of what its effects might be.

The next step is one of the most fun. Once the cannabis is ground either into a joint or a clean pipe, take a dry hit to discover the flavor. Even though the cannabis has not been lit, the taste will be incredibly pronounced.

The next thing to do after the dry hit in a cannabis tasting is to smoke. To light the joint or bowl, Podiak recommends always using hemp wick dipped in beeswax: It doesn't corrupt the taste like butane from a lighter can and allows for a cooler, cleaner smoke. Inhale slowly and gauge the flavors of the cannabis as it's exhaled.

Once everyone is tasting the cannabis, its flavor and effects will begin to unfold. This is the time to tune into how cannabis makes you feel, both in your physical body and in your mood. The taste of the joint combined with its head and body effects are a full journey.

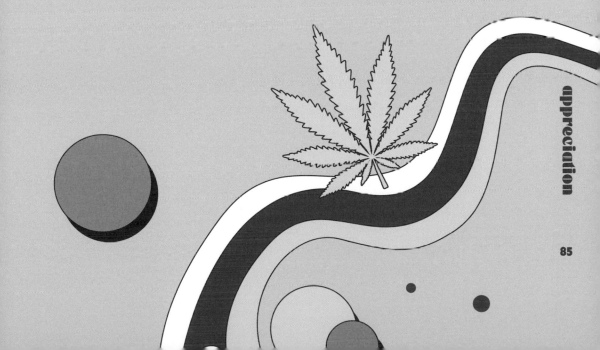

appreciation

Delectable Edibles

How It Works

When cannabis is inhaled, it is quickly released into the bloodstream through the lungs and makes its way to the brain and other parts of the body. When cannabis is ingested, THC travels through the digestive tract and is metabolized by the liver before it reaches the bloodstream. Some of the THC is converted into the more potent 11-Hydroxy-THC when it's smoked. With edibles, even more of the THC becomes converted to this other, stronger form of THC, which explains why edibles come on with more power.

Ask About the Ingredients

While many cannabis-infused food offerings out there are made with cannabis flower, leaf trim, or shake (the pieces of the flower that have fallen away from the buds), concentrates can also form a base element for edibles. There isn't much research on how different bases for edibles (cannabutter, hashish, BHO, distillate) might affect the high, but anecdotally it does feel like they make a difference.

Beyond cannabis flowers infused into something like butter, edibles can be made from kief (concentrated trichomes separated from the plant through a dry sieving) and ice-water hash (also called simply hash). Both kief and ice-water hash are methods that don't involve solvents, so they've long existed. Newer cannabinoid extraction methods often incorporate solvents. Butane hash oil (trichomes dissolved through butane) can also be used in edibles. But these days, because most people don't really like the vegetal taste that can come with cannabis flower, many store-bought edibles are made with distillate.

the delight of edibles

For me, it's a warmth, a creeping feeling of happiness from inside, a mood boost on the wings, an internal regulator capable of bringing on a positive state of mind. Cannabis edibles can be incredible tools, helping to regulate moods and dissolve body aches. They can take the botanical to all the best places in terms of its ultimate aim, homeostasis, or the steady state of internal conditions that bring about equilibrium within ourselves. The enjoyment of edibles can be powerful instruments to provide guidance toward deeper realms of our inner selves. A state of true relaxation can be achieved by using edibles with the right dosage of THC.

Due to their sedative effects, edibles are particularly useful for sleep, but they can also be put to use in smaller doses to offer balance throughout the day. Cannabis is a plant that has both a medicinal and a fun side, and because of how potent they can be, edibles cross through both worlds.

appreciation

the history of edibles

In terms of ingesting cannabis, the *Atharva Veda*, which is part of a collection of Hindu poems published in archaic Sanskrit somewhere between 2000 and 1400 BCE, has a recipe where it is speculated that the psychoactive ingredient in a drink called soma could be cannabis. Bhang is a creamy cannabis drink used in ancient India as far back as 1000 BCE, and majoon is a confection that can include honey, nuts, dried fruit, and hashish, is also an old cannabis preparation. In Ayurvedic medicine, cannabis is a trusted medicinal ingredient for a variety of health issues. In the first century, Greeks made a cannabis tincture known as kylos and throughout the Middle Ages, cannabis seeds and flowers were used in kitchens throughout Europe. *On Honorable Pleasure and Health* by Bartolomeo Platina, published in Italy in 1474 and thought to be the world's first printed cookbook, includes a recipe for "a health drink of cannabis nectar."

A few seminal texts talk about eating hashish, most notably *The Hasheesh Eater* by Fitz Hugh Ludlow, but it was the publication of a hashish fudge recipe by Alice B. Toklas that brought the concept of eating cannabis to countless people. Published in 1954, *The Alice B. Toklas Cook Book* became one of the best-selling cookbooks of all time. Toklas would later deny knowing the recipe contained hash, but its addition made the book infamous.

The history of cannabis edibles aligns with the history of cannabis cultivation in that it has strong footholds in both Holland and California. While cannabis isn't technically legal in Holland (personal use is decriminalized, however), it is tolerated and a vibrant hashish scene emerged in Amsterdam in the 1960s. The first coffeeshop, Mellow Yellow, opened in 1972 and sold hashish and cannabis-infused confections called "space cakes." In California, a woman named Mary Rathbun changed the history of marijuana's use as a medicine when she refused to stop giving people suffering from the effects of AIDS her marijuana-infused brownies, earning her the nickname Brownie Mary.

Both space cakes and brownies are desserts, and most cannabis edibles are sweets like these or gummies, but that doesn't mean they have to be. Savory edibles are also very satisfying. As cannabis edibles evolved, chefs started making dishes that were more focused on the tastes rather than diners getting as high as possible. Then cannabis started being infused in even more dishes and being incorporated into meals rather than just desserts.

Part of the evolution away from super-potent edibles is a trend toward microdoses of cannabis edibles, combined with markets opening up to consumers who may have never tried cannabis before. Many companies are making edible products with low amounts of THC that work great for people who might be interested in maintaining a low-level high throughout the day or those with a low tolerance for THC. Elise McDonough, the author of *Bong Appétit* and *The Official High Times Cannabis Cookbook*, has watched the edibles industry evolve over the years. It began as somewhat of a novelty, but she believes the future of edibles will go more toward people incorporating infused cannabis offerings as a part of their everyday healthy lifestyle. This will mean more cannabis in base ingredients such as butters or oils, or even in condiments.

appreciation

89

concentrates: the essence of the flower

Potent, powerful, and incredibly delicious, concentrates represent a paradigm shift in cannabis consumption. Concentrating and grouping cannabinoids and terpenes together to produce more potent medicine is not new; references to cannabis resin formed into hashish appear in ancient texts. What is new is the methods that producers use to create these concentrates. The rise of extraction techniques coupled with more information around the science of how cannabis works have resulted in some of the most potent, delicious "dabbable" offerings, and the ways to enjoy them have also evolved tremendously. While marijuana enthusiasts always had the option of sprinkling a bit of hashish on top of a bowl of flowers, concentrates are now products enjoyed as stand-alone offerings showcasing the finest expression of what cannabis flowers can become.

Concentrating cannabis works by removing excess plant material and keeping only the most desirable parts of the plant, the magic concoction of chemicals found in the resinous trichome heads.

When it comes to the oil for vape pens, carbon dioxide extracts are very popular. While it's a costly start-up endeavor on the business side, due to the equipment and machinery needed, the process converts trim into the cannabis oil that is the most widely sold, because it's found in most vape pens. These handheld devices rose in popularity because of their discreetness and convenience.

The Convenience of Vape Pens

the science of dabs

Extracts compile all the activated parts of the plant into the concentrated essence of what cannabis can become. As the science around how cannabis works advances, so does the science around the extraction methods. Extracts were once mostly prized for their high THC percentages, but terpenes have now entered the conversation and play a massive role in how concentrates are created and enjoyed. The type of cannabis concentrate with the most vocal fan base is made with butane and is prized for displaying a true expression of the flavors present in marijuana.

Dabs, which are generally extracts created with butane hash oil (BHO), are potent and incredibly tasty, as they amplify flavors and result in an immediate high. Dab is both a noun and a verb, standing in for the concentrate one consumes, as in "I just took a dab," as well as the action of vaporizing cannabis concentrates, or dabbing. New terms (and tools) are rapidly invented to describe the vibrant community surrounding the world of cannabis concentrates, most notably in the sphere of BHO. Taking a dab involves applying concentrate to a heated surface (a nail or quartz banger) attached to glass (a dab rig), filled with water to cool the vapor, and inhaling the concentrate.

Unlike traditional hash, the process of creating BHO doesn't rely on physical agitation to remove the resinous trichomes. Instead, it dissolves them, and the ways of removing the residual solvent determine the style of extract. Butane is highly flammable, and creating BHO without the proper tools, or open blasting, can result in deadly explosions. To do it properly, extractors need to invest in a closed-loop extraction system.

Another helpful cannabis concentrate term to become acquainted with is nug run, which describes high-quality concentrates made with flowers instead of trim, the leafy parts of the plant that are removed as cannabis is trimmed into flower buds (also called nugs).

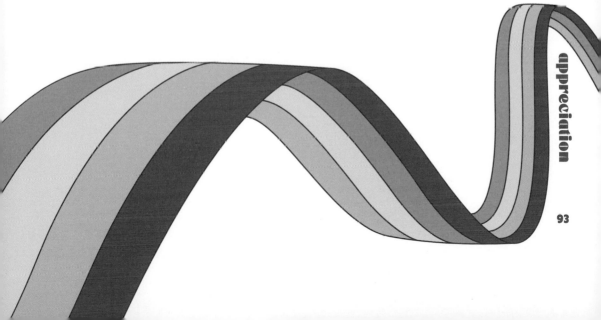

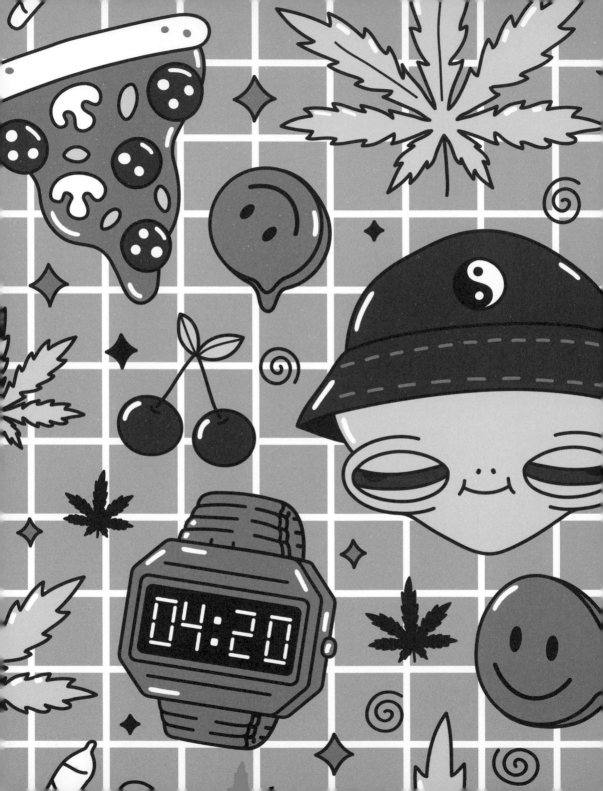

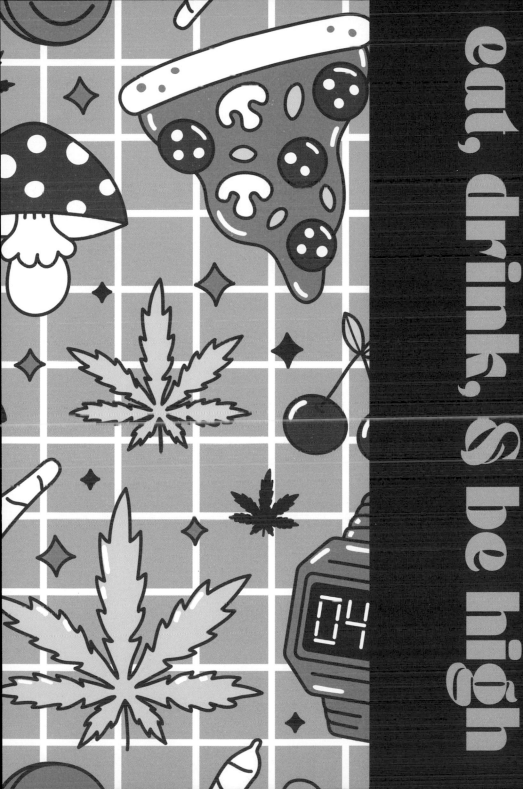

eat, drink, & be high

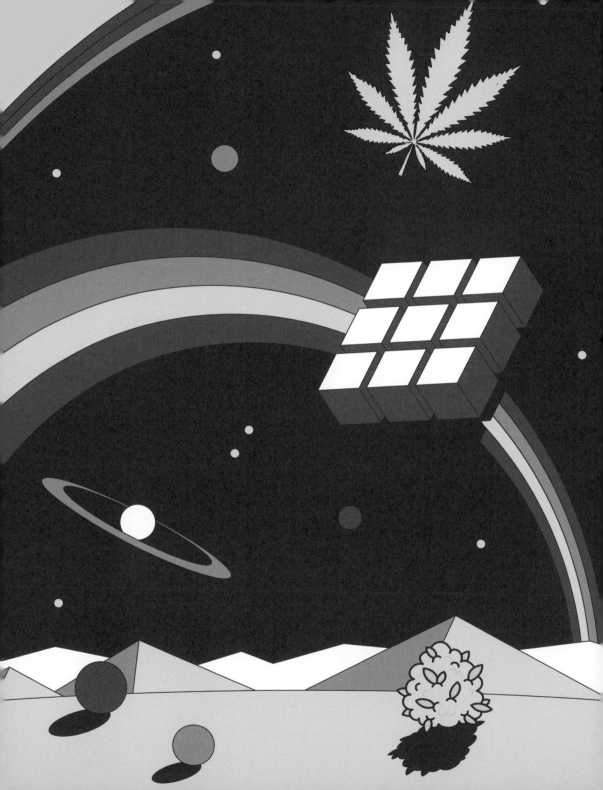

cannabis as a superfood

Known for their high nutritional value, superfoods are considered to be especially beneficial for health and well-being. Often plant-based, but also including some fish and dairy, superfood is a marketing word to describe foods containing various nutrients, such as antioxidants and healthy fats. A key to finding them comes with phytochemicals, or the chemicals in plants responsible for deep colors and smells.

Think blueberries, salmon, kale, and acai. Juicing cannabis was popularized by Dr. William Courtney, founder of Cannabis International, a resource organization for the dietary and medicinal uses of cannabis. Akin to daily fatty acids and essential amino acids, Courtney believes there should be "minimum daily requirements established to guide worldwide adoption of raw cannabis as the single most important dietary element." The benefits of juicing allow for the vitamins and enzymes in raw fruits and vegetables to rapidly enter the bloodstream and promote health. Viewing cannabis as a superfood falls in line with both its preventative and restorative qualities.

"Cannabis is a unique functional food that, if used in its natural state daily, provides benefits in excess of nutrition," Courtney wrote in the cannabis trade publication, *Treating Yourself*, describing his trials juicing cannabis for patients in Mendocino and Humboldt Counties.

cannabis pairings

Curated cannabis experiences coupled with food and wine pairings are rising in popularity as more and more people become comfortable enjoying cannabis in a group setting. While experiencing culinary cannabis in a restaurant is still in the initial development stages, private pop-up events in places with legal cannabis are expanding. These events play an important role in building a community around a shared interest and can offer intimate glimpses into the lives of the farmers who cultivate cannabis flowers. The gatherings also provide participants with a further understanding of the botanical elements of marijuana. Chefs can incorporate different parts of the plant, such as the leaves or even pickled pollen sacs from male plants, into the meal.

Pot-infused pop-ups take on many forms. Some of them use the events as educational opportunities to demo different methods for infusing cannabis into food. Others skip the infused cuisine altogether, instead pairing courses with compatible tastes in cultivars smoked at the table. All look to cannabis as another ingredient in the kitchen to add to fine dining's overall sensory experience.

cannabis meets culinary tastemakers

Rachel Burkons, who along with her brother, Holden Jagger, runs the cannabis hospitality company Altered Plates, is an educator, activist, and self-coined "bong vivant." In 2019, Altered Plates hosted a dinner and educational event at the James Beard House in New York City. The James Beard Foundation continues to set the stage for innovations in the culinary world, and the dinner marked a critical moment for the acceptance of cannabis into the modern restaurant world. Its success lay in pairing hemp with other high-quality ingredients and incorporating other elements that one might expect at a James Beard-recognized restaurant experience, including expert wine pairings and impeccable service.

"Cannabis can bring an entirely new experience to something as universal as a wonderful meal," Burkons says. "Not only does cannabis provide a relaxing, enjoyable high, but it can enhance the flavors in a dish, and it can change the energy in the room."

Many have likely heard that marijuana can give you the "munchies," but Burkons says that the simple fact of the matter is that food tastes great when you're high. Cannabis dinner parties also have a different vibe than alcohol-fueled events, she says.

"There's a lot of laughter and connection happening, but it feels more intentional and sincere than the events and spaces where alcohol is the choice social lubricant."

eat, drink, & be high

99

There are several ways to incorporate cannabis into a dining experience, from infused dinners and drinks to cannabis tasting sessions with food pairings. When Burkons is hosting an event, she's hyper-focused on elevating the presentation of the star ingredient within the event or dinner setting. "From elegant joints passed alongside canapés to floral arrangements adorned with a cannabis leaf or flower, every element of a high-dining experience can feature cannabis in a different, unique, and exciting way for the guest," she says.

The meal menu at the Beard House included a carrot-tangerine soup with smoked parsnips, Spanish jamón, and a honey infused with terpenes pulled from other plants that Jagger reconstructed to duplicate the profile of Black Lime, a boutique Northern California cultivar with hints of both black pepper and lime. A salad included delicate young hemp shoots amid a bed of more traditional leafy greens.

Like all fine dining, the key to elevated cannabis cuisine is in the pairings. The hope is to create perfect harmony by incorporating the taste profiles present in the cannabis flower with complementary flavors in food and wine. At Altered Plates, Burkons and Jagger take the strategies they would use to match wine and food and use them for pairing cannabis with their dishes. "Pairing wine and food is something we understand as being built on a harmonious expression of flavors, and it's no different with cannabis," Burkons explains. "Because each cannabis variety has its own unique flavors and aromas, seeking that same balance when pairing with a dish is essential."

Her expert advice for cannabis pairings with food is to match contrasting flavors. "In terms of finding harmony and balance in a pairing, that generally means one of two things: pairing like flavors with like, or pairing contrasting flavors from opposite ends of the flavor wheel," she says. "The most effective and exciting pairings tend to take two contrasting flavors—sweet and spice, earthy and citrusy, tropical and herbal—and match them against each other, but sometimes playing up a note in a dish with a cannabis variety that matches its flavor profile is highly effective as well."

It's one thing to pair food and cannabis or food and wine, but it's another to appropriately pair all three.

"Bringing together all three elements is another challenge that requires a keen focus on balance," Burkons says. "Finding that combination between like and dissimilar flavors across the palate becomes key, and the order in which you taste specific things might be important. For example, we frequently tell a guest to finish a course with its cannabis pairing, so perhaps the wine would be paired with the dish as the guest eats, and the cannabis can act as a digestif or vice versa. There really is so much to play with in terms of big, interesting flavors in cannabis, and there is so much to experiment with."

When it comes to an infused meal, a crucial element also comes in the dosage, as the last thing that hosts want is for diners to get uncomfortably high. Coreen Carroll is the chef behind the

Cannaisseur Series, a winner of the Netflix cooking competition *Cooked with Cannabis*, and co-author of the book *Edibles: Small Bites for the Modern Cannabis Kitchen*. She says a critical component of being a cannabis chef is making sure diners stay in their comfort zone.

"It's important to remember it's not all about just getting high," she says. "All of my events, whether for a private party or for public events, are meant to be shared between everyone from the novice to the occasional user to the experienced consumer. Therefore, it's important to offer [cannabis] while educating about how to use it properly, depending on your comfort level. I am a cannabis chef, and it is my responsibility to guide you through a cannabis dining experience that you can enjoy and remember." Carroll sees her ticketed events and private pop-ups as providing a crucial space for cannabis enthusiasts to gather and explore the plant together in a way that wasn't possible before, due to marijuana's illegal associations. The plant, she says, brings together people of all different backgrounds. "Cannabis has become the wine accoutrement to dining," she says. "Unlike alcohol, cannabis has the ability to bring people together, especially when being able to share and pass a joint. This simple motion connects a large room of consumers. When we all take part in tasting, learning, and feeling the instant effects, it allows humans to communicate more openly and freely."

At her events, the experience takes place at communal tables to help facilitate sharing and communication. Carroll often combines infused elements alongside intermezzo cannabis joints between courses.

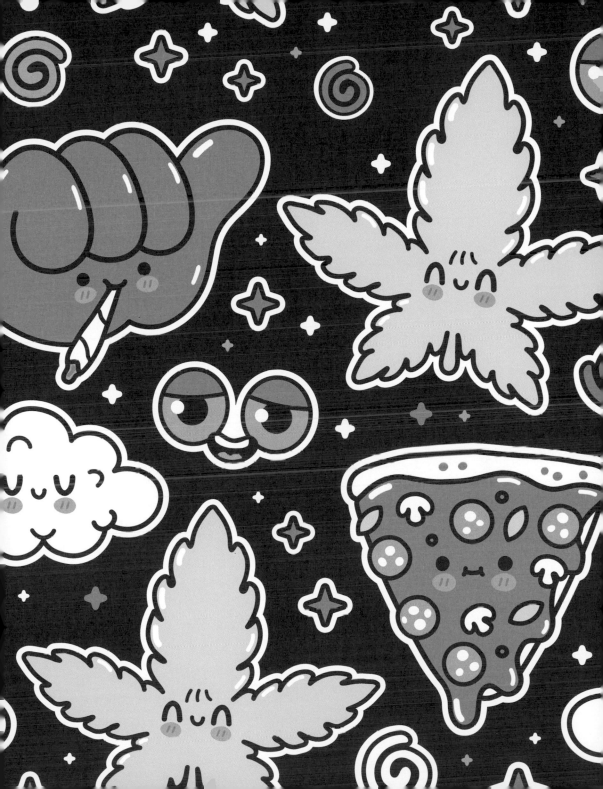

Any good cannabis dining experience aims to guide diners through the meal in a way that allows them to feel a bit stoned, but still also comfortable in their surroundings. To do this, Carroll uses the effects of cannabis as a guide and offers joint pairings in between courses. She starts with a more elevated head high from a bright, uplifting flower on the sativa-side of the spectrum, then moves on to the high-CBD flowers to balance the elevation of THC and ends with buds from the indica side of cannabis that result in more of a high felt in the body rather than the mind. Carroll infuses the food courses with only non-psychoactive parts of the plant, including THCA, CBDA, cannabis leaves, or terpenes.

"I like infusing CBD and offering CBD flower joints in the middle of my events; it helps reset the crowd and keeps any overconsumption of THC at bay," she says of the cannabinoid's ability to counteract some of the negative effects of feeling too high. "CBD allows for a longer and more enjoyable experience."

the herb somm

Named by *Wine Enthusiast* magazine as one of its Top 40 Under 40 tastemakers, Jamie Evans brings a decade of wine experience into her work in cannabis hospitality. As the founder of cannabis and lifestyle brand The Herb Somm, Evans approaches tasting cannabis in the same way that a sommelier comes to tasting wine.

"As it turns out, there are many similarities when it comes to wine and cannabis," she says. "Not only do these two categories share similar aroma and flavor profiles, but they are both terroir-expressive plants."

Evans explains that, like grapes, cannabis takes on a sense of "place and practice."

"Depending on where the cannabis is grown, strains express unique characteristics based on the microclimates that the plant comes from," she says. "Much like vineyard owners care for their grapevines, cannabis farmers also believe that terroir is so much more than just weather and soil. As a farmer, they're a part of the terroir. Every growing method and practice they use plays an essential role in the plant's well-being."

Evans hosts a private dining club in San Francisco called Thursday Infused. The events, often held within homes, also act as brand introductions, as producers can talk to guests about their products. This exchange creates transparency in the product's

eat, drink, & be high

creation, allowing diners to meet brand representatives and farmers face-to-face.

"One of the most incredible things about cannabis is it brings people together," she says. "I've also always found that cannabis is more approachable and relatable when combined with food and beverages."

Following the steps for a successful wine tasting, diners evaluate cannabis first by its looks, then by its smell, followed by its taste and effects.

"As we do in the wine world, we can interpret the unique characteristics of cannabis by training our nose and palates to recognize the nuances between each strain," Evans says. "By analyzing terpene profiles, we can pair cannabis with food and wine. Cannabis is also an incredible gourmet ingredient that has the ability to enhance the dining experience, just like wine."

Smelling cannabis lights up olfactory zones and provides a guide map to how the experience can go. Tasting marijuana reveals its structure against the salty, sour, sweet, and bitter tastes the tongue can detect. Both properly smelling and tasting cannabis are associated with an understanding of its terpenes, the organic compounds that create aroma and flavors in cannabis and other plants. To put this all together in line with wine tastings, Evans places aromatic plants containing terpenes, such as lavender, citrus, black pepper, and pine needles, within wineglasses. Evans learned this technique when she studied viticulture at Cal Poly in San Luis Obispo from a sensory evaluation teacher who built an aroma bar. "This practice immensely helped me learn how to decipher a wine's profile by training the nose and palate to recognize different smells and tastes," she says.

Using the same wineglass technique, Evans invites guests at her events to take in the aroma profiles of cannabis and develop their own "herbal palate."

"Use your nose to smell through different ingredients that are often used to describe cannabis's aromas and flavors," she advises. "For example, put slices of lemon, lime, and grapefruit in separate wineglasses. Close your eyes, smell the ingredients, and try to remember what each different citrus fruit smells like. Next, taste the ingredients and savor the flavor on your palate. What you're smelling and tasting are terpenes."

When enjoying a little weed with your wine, a general rule to follow is to pair light and energizing strains with white wines, while pairing bold and relaxing cultivars with red wines.

"And when it comes to rosé, you can really get creative because, in my view, rosé is one of the most versatile wines to pair with cannabis," she says. "There are many combinations that work well, which is something that we also observe when pairing rosé with food."

eat, drink, & be high

cannabis cocktails

Cannabis cocktails are high on the list of luxury items in the cannabis space because of their association with the luxuriant and opulent worlds that cocktail culture occupies. Mixing drinks was once considered a simple act, but it has been elevated to an art form with bartenders becoming "mixologists" and serving drinks in elegant stemware within lavish locations.

Pairing cannabis and spirits is a master class in blending flavors.

"Different varietals and cultivars have different aromas," says Warren Bobrow, author of *Cannabis Cocktails, Mocktails & Tonics*. "When you decarb [cannabis flower], the terpenes become really exemplary in the craft cocktail world."

When he works with infused spirits for a cannabis cocktail, Bobrow sticks within the darker color range of alcohol because the infusion in a lighter-colored spirit makes the drink turn an unpleasant brown shade. He likes to infuse spirits like scotch, cognac, and Armagnac; he also works with Madeira, a fortified wine, and Belgian lambics.

"I love the Belgian cherry beers, the sour cherry ales, they're amazing to infuse," he says. "All you have to do is infuse maybe three ounces and then mix that three ounces back into the twelve-ounce bottle and you have a perfectly infused twelve-ounce beer."

Beyond infusing the alcohol itself, he often also infuses other elements that go into a cocktail. For example, during his appearance on *VICE Live*, Bobrow roasted blood oranges with angostura bitters and combined this with barrel bourbon and a ginger beer syrup infused with 2,500 milligrams of THC, so the drink was one hundred milligrams per fluid ounce. To be clear, one hundred milligrams in a glass is an incredibly strong infusion. More novice edible cannabis consumers find their edge of comfort at around ten milligrams.

"When I do private parties, [the guests] know what they're getting into," he explains of his heavy-hitting drinks. "And I do say, always, never have more than one drink per hour because everyone is different, and what affects me might not affect you, but it might destroy the person next to you, so you have to start slow. It's like Thai food. You don't go to a Thai food restaurant and order five-star spicy. I mean, crazy people do, but I don't recommend it. With cannabis cocktails, you want to start with a very little bit."

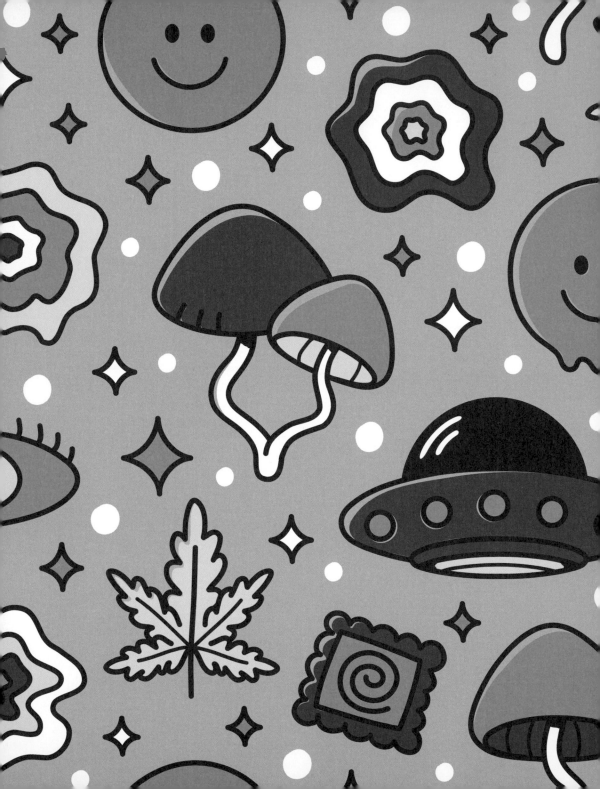

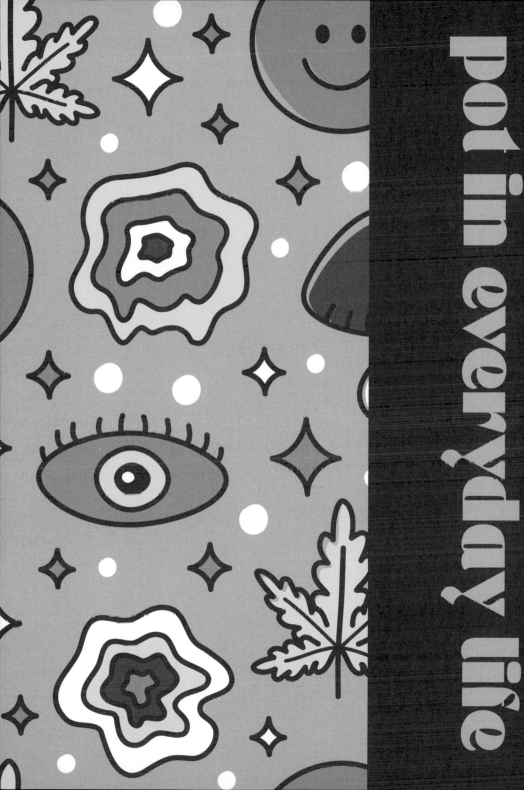

pot in everyday life

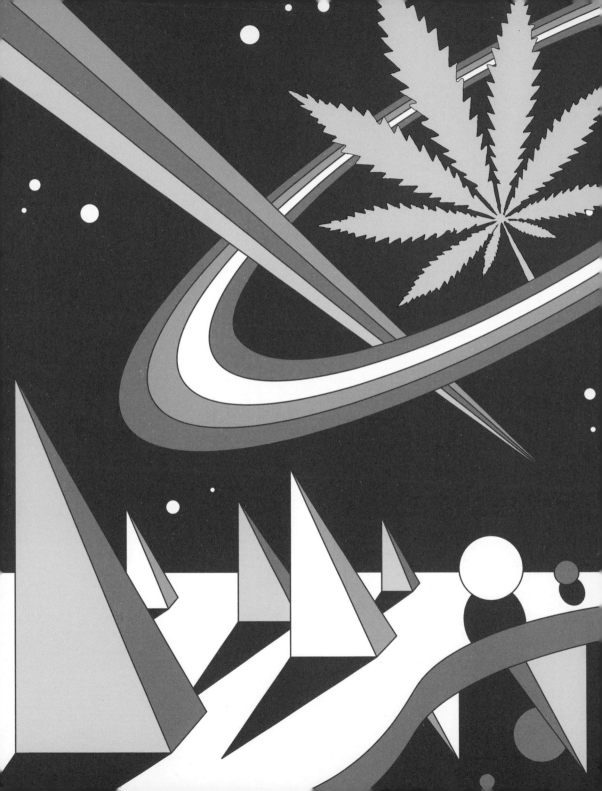

a leaf of luxury

It's a beautiful thing that cannabis can open itself up to the world again. Cannabis is breaking free from negative associations and finding proper acknowledgment as one of the finest agricultural products on Earth, worthy of the highest praise and enjoyed with the appropriate reverence. While proper legalization should mean that cannabis can be obtained at a similar price point to beer to offer a healthier alternative to the common intoxicant, there's no reason why premium flowers can't also go for a premium price. Luxury products purchased to enhance the enjoyment of weed showcase that the humble herb is a genuinely desirable commodity.

Cannabis concentrates are some of the priciest ways to enjoy the botanical. A gram of live resin from a premium producer can easily go for more than a hundred dollars, so it makes sense that many high-end items have been created to appreciate and savor concentrates. Taking a dab at the right temperature is the height of the cannabis-tasting experience. Vaporized in such a way that the terpenes are perfectly preserved, dabs unveil the essence of the flower and put all of marijuana's aromas and tastes on a kaleidoscopic display of deliciousness.

In the luxury space, a lot of the importance is within the act of being seen. Designer Alexander Wang's Fall 2016 collection incorporated cannabis prints in a few key places and helped form the idea of cannabis couture. In terms of fashion, cannabis influences are showing up on the runway in clothing as well as jewelry and accessories. Vivienne Westwood has included a cannabis leaf print dress in a runway show and Jacquie Aiche, a jeweler with celebrity admirers whose work appears in high-end shops such as Saks Fifth Avenue, designed a whole line of jewelry dedicated to the leaf. Called Sweet Leaf, the collection includes a 14K yellow-gold bracelet with a diamond-encrusted cannabis leaf shape surrounded by pavé diamonds, priced at nearly $6,000.

The makers behind Ras Boss jewelry take the concept of cannabis jewelry even further by dipping real cannabis leaves and flowers in 24K gold. These pieces are wearable cannabis art. The hoop earrings are crafted from a curling cannabis leaf and the necklaces are buds that have been dipped in gold and resemble gold nuggets in their organic shapes. Many of the nug necklaces are also studded with other jewels. An OG Kush nug with sapphire and opal is priced at $780 and a nug with a string of amethyst, emeralds, and a diamond is $2,200.

Cannabis branding for flowers and edibles is also looking a lot more lux lately. By adopting minimalistic designs, brands are looking to influence cannabis tastemakers and set themselves apart in an increasingly crowded market. To do so, they've dedicated a lot of time to the presentation and packaging. Consumers who are already fashionable in other areas bring fashion into their cannabis purchases and only want to be seen puffing the best.

While Barneys New York's attempt at selling high-end cannabis accessories (including a $1,100 bong at an LA in-store boutique called the High End) ultimately ended when the department store, which once reigned in the world of high fashion, shut down for good in 2020, the concept of upscale smoking accessories in high-end shopping locations has likely not seen its final days, as new cannabis markets continue to open.

cannabis in ritual

Cannabis, both as hemp and as a psychoactive substance, has historical footholds in forms of rituals dating all the way back to the ancient world. During funeral rituals, the Scythians, a nomadic people who migrated from Central Asia across to Southern Russia and the Ukraine in the eighth and seventh centuries BCE, would fill a pit with hot rocks, make a tent over the pit, and then throw hemp seed on the hot stones and inhale "such a vapor as no Grecian vapor-bath can exceed; the Scythians, delighted, shout for joy," the Greek historian Herodotus writes in his book *Histories* around 425 BCE. A 2,500-year-old Siberian "ice princess" was buried with cannabis, and wooden bowls excavated from a tomb dating back to a 2,500-year-old cemetery in Western China bear traces of THC.

medicine melodies

One of the appeals of cannabis is how present it can make you feel. Based out of Los Angeles, Rachel Dugas offers cannabis-enhanced sound baths at yoga studios and private locations. Dugas found herself turning toward mindfulness practices partially through her work for a cannabis vaporizer company, Firefly, then later decided to pursue a certification in sound, voice, and music in the healing arts at the California Institute of Integral Studies.

"I started learning about medicine melodies, which are more associated with the ayahuasca plant, but basically, it's the idea that you can channel melodies of the plant and the consciousness of the plant," she says. "And then I realized, 'Oh! I'm already doing this with weed. Other people want to do this too.'"

Dugas explains that relaxation is a crucial element in absorbing a sound bath's healing powers; but it takes a while to get relaxed, to still your mind and stop your thoughts, and cannabis can help.

"It puts you in an immediate relaxed space," she says. "I think the healing properties of the plant make it conducive to other healing experiences."

marijuana mindfulness

Dee Dussault has made a name for herself by publicly offering yoga classes enhanced by cannabis since 2009. She wrote a book, *Ganja Yoga*, which was published in 2017, and started a ganja yoga teacher training course to instruct others.

"We start off with what I call a stoner social," Dussault says of her yoga classes. "So the first half an hour we're consuming together. And then we begin the yoga with meditation and mindfulness, so people are invited to become aware of their high and feel how the cannabis impacts the rest of the yoga session."

Dussault explains that yoga works well with cannabis because it makes people more aware of their bodies, relaxes the body, and has pain-relieving qualities such as the ability to combat inflammation.

"I use cannabis with my yoga and meditation with my personal use as well as with my classes," she says. "I'm a regular cannabis user, so I use it throughout the day outside of a yoga context. What I like about using it is that it gives me a chance to sort of step outside the business of my moment and take a little retreat or respite for myself. I'm more mindful. I try not to use cannabis [while I'm] on my phone or, you know, scrolling Instagram. It gives me a chance to just sort of tune into myself and ground into myself. In a way, it's a kind of yoga practice. I mean, I'm obviously not doing poses, but it's an opportunity for me to connect myself, which is really what yoga is all about."

Jessica Dugan, who went through Dussault's Ganja Yoga teacher training in 2018 and founded a cannabis retreat for industry professionals called Reflections, agrees that cannabis helps bridge the gap between mind and body.

"Cannabis heightens our awareness, which makes the practitioner more aware of how they feel in their body, what their body is wanting movement-wise [which is] sometimes no movement at all," she says. "Sometimes, those of us who have a lot of pain benefit from cannabis as an analgesic because reducing the pain helps us get onto the mat in the first place. It makes the practice accessible. The combination of breath and movement medicine is already so beneficial for our nervous system and emotions. By adding cannabis to the practice, we are also activating receptors in the emotional processing center, limbic brain, to further support unwinding from our days and whatever emotions our bodies might be holding on to."

Duyan's use of cannabis in her own life is a profoundly reflective act, one that she uses sparingly as a tool to discover her own thoughts and feelings.

"When I'm really stuck and need insight, I open my altar, make prayers, and ask cannabis for support with proper reverence," she says. "Imbibing cannabis in the ceremonial space has made room for more purposeful or spiritual conversations."

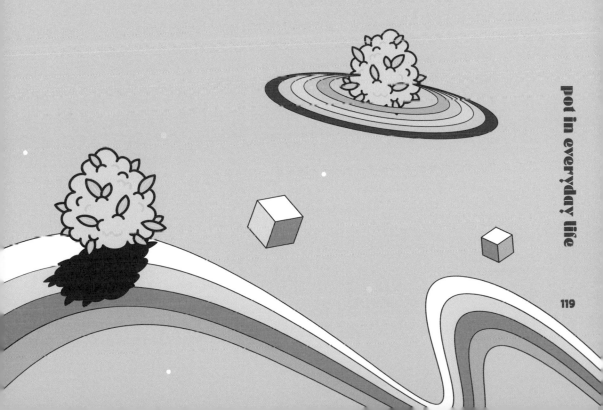

cannabis & creative expression

Our relationship with the cannabis plant often fuels creative self-expression. For many creative people, cannabis provides the necessary fuel to express themselves in this world through its ability to bring us into different mindsets. Cannabis is also now an integral part of the wider culture. Where cannabis enthusiasts were once only shown as lazy stoners, portrayals of marijuana consumers are finally getting more nuanced and truthful in showing that many different types of people have a special relationship with this plant. The truth is, no other plant that has been so vilified still has so many loyal fans willing to turn out in droves to enjoy it together and celebrate their fandom.

puff, pass & paint

Paint and sip, the idea of art nights involving wine, is a business that has grown so large in recent years that it's expanded from single-outlet operations into franchises. Taking that business concept further is an art event

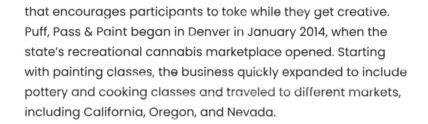

that encourages participants to toke while they get creative. Puff, Pass & Paint began in Denver in January 2014, when the state's recreational cannabis marketplace opened. Starting with painting classes, the business quickly expanded to include pottery and cooking classes and traveled to different markets, including California, Oregon, and Nevada.

The way that Puff, Pass & Paint classes work is by welcoming participants to bring their own stash. Everyone present at the private events must be twenty-one, the legal age for adult-use cannabis consumption. Art supplies, snacks, and drinks are provided and people work at communal tables with assistance from art instructors.

"Cannabis brings everyone together in a way that I think a lot of things don't," Keyes says. "In our classes we see a wide age range with people from all over the place, of all different backgrounds, which I think is a really neat thing."

glass art

Glass art started with glassblowers making pipes and bongs to enjoy cannabis flowers, but it evolved immensely in the mid-2000s; as the processes to create cannabis concentrates became more refined, so too did the glass used to enjoy concentrates. The pipes explicitly used for cannabis concentrates are called dab rigs, and creating this form of glass art sent glass-collecting into new realms in terms of both demand and price.

Based in Washington State, Mothership Glass set the stage for high-end glass-collecting when it began in 2013. Mothership crafts functional glass art using techniques that incorporate intricate detail and elements of sacred geometry, a belief that ascribes symbolic and religious meanings to geometric shapes.

Beyond dab rigs, glass art in the concentrate community also includes decorative carb caps, an accessory that creates suction when placed on top of a nail or a quartz banger (the areas where

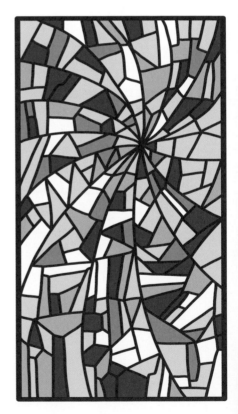

the concentrate is applied). Dab tools scoop up and spread the concentrate to the nail or quartz banger and dab pearls (small marble-like balls designed to spin around inside of quartz bangers to improve vaporization). There's also glass art that's purely decorative, with artistically created pendants worn on necklaces that are affectionately known as "heady pendies."

cannabis photography

As weed becomes legal in more places, photographers have more and more access to material to shoot, rather than being limited by the need for secrecy with illegal plants. And the ways they are shooting cannabis are changing, with many contemporary cannabis photographers using a technique called focus stacking. This 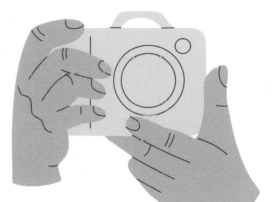 digital photography tool combines multiple images taken at different focuses to provide images at the highest possible definition. These macro shots look much like underwater scenes or alien lifeforms. They depict the trichomes, fine outgrowths on the flowers, at scales imperceptible to the naked human eye. Focus-stacking techniques can involve dozens or hundreds of images. The method can be used to zoom in extremely close to look at the trichome "hairs" and the resinous heads up top containing cannabinoids and terpenes, or depict the flower's fullness from a bit further back so viewers can get lost in all the colors and depth of the blossoms. Videography also allows some advanced photographers to catch the plant's image at all angles and zoom in and out as the flower spins in place.

Cannabis photography is not only a form of creative artistic expression, but a way to demystify the plant and spread knowledge about the varied ways by which the flower expresses itself.

social smoke lounges

Cannabis is now legal for those over the age of twenty-one in many states across the nation. But cannabis enthusiasts often don't get to celebrate the same rites of passage as those who reach the minimum drinking age. Even though marijuana is legal in more places than ever before, smoking lounges offering safe places to consume cannabis are still few and far between.

A city that has embraced smoking lounges is the one where they got their start, San Francisco. There you will find enough cannabis dispensaries with lounges so close to each other that they could be visited in succession in much the same way as a pub crawl. It feels a bit like visiting the coffeeshops in

Amsterdam. Each shop has its own unique feel and appeals that range from what kinds of smoking accessories are offered to other amenities such as comfortable seating and free hot tea.

In the 1970s and '80s, Dennis Peron had already been busted for selling pot multiple times. Still, he continued to sell cannabis out of his living room in San Francisco's Castro District, inviting everyone he met to join in what would become known as the legendary philosophical salon and marijuana marketplace called the Big Top. Originally from the Bronx, Peron arrived in San Francisco in 1969 after serving in the Air Force in Vietnam during the Tet Offensive. The Big Top gatherings would eventually evolve into a cannabis consumption-friendly restaurant space downstairs called the Island. Then, a personal tragedy would spur Peron to open the first public marijuana dispensary in the US, but it was also much more than that; it was a welcome open environment where people were invited to freely consume cannabis.

The second iteration of Peron's shop, the Cannabis Buyers' Club, was a 2,000-square-foot space located above a bar on the corner of Church and Market Streets that opened in 1994. With ten-foot-tall ceilings in the main room displaying a massive swath of rainbow flags, crystals, and brightly colored stained glass

in the windows, the
club fulfilled critical
social and emotional needs.
Here, patients suffering from
the crippling effects of the AIDS crisis
could purchase their medication and
emerge from the isolation of their illnesses.

Peron's longtime companion, Jonathan West, had passed away
from AIDS in 1990, and Peron had seen how much cannabis had
helped West ease his pain and restore his appetite. After a bust
when police entered their home and treated the dying man with
extreme disregard, Peron envisioned a place where West could
have gone to socialize and be among friends. Not only did the
Cannabis Buyers' Club become a place to find marijuana, it
became a community gathering space for people who had lost
their jobs, their housing, and their friends when they became ill.

Consumption spaces set the scene for new experiences and
helped familiarize people with the different ways in which
cannabis can be enjoyed. Employees in these spaces can make

recommendations for choosing cannabis flowers and help people learn how to enjoy cannabis at a rate that allows them to achieve a comfortable high.

They are also important gathering places to foster cannabis culture, either by trying out new smoking devices on loan or by socializing with others within the space. The decor of these clubs helps to allow for different experiences. Some are opulently decorated like historic speakeasy lounges of the jazz era, while others are effortlessly sleek and contemporary. As a part of the older medical marijuana holistic wellness model, lounges can also provide a space for communal activities such as yoga or game nights. One lounge in San Francisco that I've visited resembles a sports bar with lots of TVs playing the game and makes a great alternative to visiting a bar during significant sporting events.

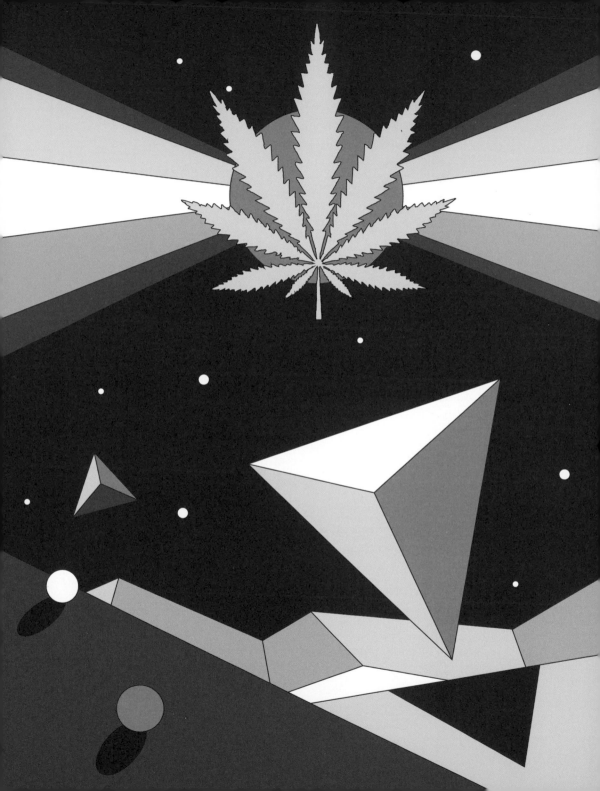

glossary

Activated isolates: A crystalline solid or powder that contains an isolated cannabinoid.

Anandamide: A cannabinoid that is generated within the body.

Bhang: A creamy cannabis drink used in ancient India as far back as 1000 BCE.

Body-high: The effects of cannabis that are felt within the body as opposed to the mind.

Broad-spectrum: A product that still contains most of the naturally-occurring cannabinoids and terpenes, but not THC.

Butane hash oil (BHO): A concentrate created when the trichomes are dissolved through butane.

Cannabichromene (CBC): A cannabinoid that has potent anti-inflammatory effects and treats pain.

Cannabidiol (CBD): The second most prevalent cannabinoid found in cannabis. This cannabinoid doesn't make people feel "stoned" or intoxicated and can alleviate some of the adverse effects of feeling too high.

Cannabigerol (CBG): A cannabinoid that is the building block for what later becomes THC and CBD.

Cannabinol (CBN): A sedative cannabinoid that THC turns into as it ages.

Caryophyllene: Also found in black pepper, caryophyllene has a spicy scent and activates cannabinoid receptors within peripheral tissues, the parts of the body that act as a response to a change in the environment, such as skin.

CBD isolate: Products that only contain CBD.

Charas: Hand-rolled resin, this is the original concentrate. Rubbing live cannabis flowers at the peak of ripeness will result in the transfer of the sticky THC-laden resin.

Chemotypes: The chemical makeup of different plants. In cannabis it's cannabinoids and terpenes that make up a plant's chemical fingerprint.

Cola: The tight buds that form at the tip of the cannabis stem.

Cultivars: Short for "cultivated variety," this means a plant produced by selective breeding.

Dab: Both a noun and a verb, a "dab" is the concentrate one consumes, and "dabbing" is the process of vaporizing cannabis concentrates.

Dab pearls: Small, marble-like balls designed to spin around inside of quartz bangers to improve vaporization.

Decarboxylation: A chemical reaction that occurs when you add heat to the flowers either through the act of lighting a joint or bowl, vaporizing, or applying heat for crafting edibles with an oven or slow cooker. Decarboxylation "activates" the chemical elements of cannabis.

Dioecious: Plants that naturally reproduce through wind carrying pollen from the male plants to the flowers on female plants.

Distillate: An odorless and flavorless substance concentrate that's an increasingly popular option for vape pens.

Dutch coffeeshops: Establishments in the Netherlands where cannabis for personal consumption is tolerated.

Endocannabinoid system: A full-body signaling network that includes receptor sites CB1 and CB2, configured to bind to cannabinoids and terpenes.

Endocannabinoids: Cannabinoids produced by the human body.

Entourage effect: The harmony between how the various components of the cannabis plant, cannabinoids, and terpenes work together.

Fan leaves: The large, fingered leaves on the cannabis plant.

Full-spectrum: A product that has most of the naturally occurring cannabinoids and terpenes in the plant, including THC.

Genetics: In cannabis this term is used to describe the genetic makeup of plants, the genotype. In other words, the cultivars that were bred to create a new type of marijuana. It's also a sort of shorthand for seeds and clones.

Genotypes: The genetic makeup of plants.

Hashish/hash: A concentrate created by using water and ice to agitate the trichomes, which are sieved into porous bags (also called ice-water hash).

Hügelkultur: A horticultural technique of creating a mound with decaying wood and filling it with compostable materials to create a rich soil, which is then added to year over year.

Humulene: Found in hops, basil, coriander, cloves, ginseng, and ginger, humulene has woodsy, earthy flavors and possesses formidable anti-inflammatory properties.

Indicas: Short, squat plants with broad leaves, shorter flowering times, and powerful sedative effects.

Kief: A concentrate created by running cannabis flowers and/or trim over a mesh grate to sieve apart the trichomes.

Landrace varieties: Cannabis that has not been hybridized and imparts the unique tastes of place; the oldest, purest cannabis and the foundational building blocks of marijuana.

Larfy: A slang term for smaller immature buds.

Limonene: The terpene present in citrus fruits.

Linalool: Also found in lavender, linalool can produce sedative calming effects and reduce agitation.

Live resin: Cannabis concentrates crafted from fresh frozen material rather than material that has been dried and cured.

Majoon: A confection that can include honey, nuts, dried fruit, and hashish.

Myrcene: The most common terpene in cannabis, it has a synergistic effect with THC that enhances its sedative properties. It is also in lemongrass, thyme, and mangoes.

Nail: A metal object attached to a dab rig where concentrate is applied.

NORML: National Organization for the Reform of Marijuana Laws, founded in 1970 in Washington, DC.

Nug run: High-quality concentrates made with cannabis flowers instead of trim.

Pheno hunt/selection: The search for the best characteristics among cultivars, the best phenotypes. Breeders select phenotypes for particular attributes such as resin production, aromas, or looks.

Phenotypes: A genetic term that breaks down to the physical characteristics a plant expresses in relation to its environment. It is a term often misused to describe the differing genetic expression of cannabis plants from seed.

Phytocannabinoids: Cannabinoids produced by plants.

Pinene: The terpene in pine needles, rosemary, basil, and cannabis cultivars like Dutch Treat and Jack Herer. It's the terpene that is most prevalent in nature in both coniferous trees and other plants, and studies have shown it can enhance memory and cognition.

Quartz banger: An alternative to a nail, these are buckets made of quartz, meant for dabbing.

Rosin: A newer type of cannabis concentrate that works by applying heat and pressure to cannabis flowers to squeeze out sticky resin.

Ruderalis: Small plants that possess the ability to flower based on the plant's maturity rather than the cycle of light or "auto-flowering."

Sativas: Tall plants with thin leaves, long flowering times, and uplifting highs.

Sauce and diamonds: These BHO extracts resemble what they sound like in either drippy, sticky material filled with terpenes or pure cannabinoids formed into hard crystallized nuggets resembling diamonds. They are heated to 90 to 100 degrees Fahrenheit and do not require a vacuum purge because the process involves cannabinoids in crystallized form and their natural separation from terpenes through a chemical process called recrystallization. These are not crafted with cannabis that has been traditionally dried and cured, but from fresh plants that have been frozen, all to better preserve and isolate terpenes.

Schwazzing: A growing technique of extreme defoliation, where 100 percent of the fan leaves are removed from the plant during different times in the flowering cycle.

Shake: Pieces of the flower that fall away from the buds.

Shatter: A BHO extract that is heated to 68 to 115 degrees Fahrenheit with a high-pressure vacuum purge that takes on the hardened translucent ambers and golds of glass.

Solventless hash: Cannabis extracts created without the use of chemical solvents such as butane or propane.

Sugar leaves: So named because of the sugary coating of trichomes they receive at the end of the flowering phase.

Terpenes: Found in the oily resin of cannabis, these hydrocarbon compounds make up the aromatic oils of a wide variety of plants and are responsible for the tastes, smells, and effects of marijuana.

Terpenoids: Terpenes with an additional chemical component, usually oxygen.

Terpinolene: A terpene in apples, lilacs, nutmeg, and cumin. Its scents pull from all over the spectrum, with a bit of woodsy earth combined with citrusy pine notes.

Tetrahydrocannabinol (THC): The most well-recognized cannabinoid, it's the one that's primarily responsible for the psychoactive effects of cannabis, the "high."

Tetrahydrocannabivarin (THCV): A rare cannabinoid that acts as an appetite suppressant.

Titrate: To measure and balance the effects of marijuana.

Trichomes: The resinous, microscopic, mushroom-looking heads found on cannabis flowers, where cannabinoids concentrate.

Trim: The leafy parts of the plant that are removed as cannabis is trimmed into flower buds.

Wax/budder: BHO extracts that are yellowish in color, but also opaque and look like butter. They are heated to 110 to 120 degrees Fahrenheit with a low-pressure vacuum purge.

glossary

135

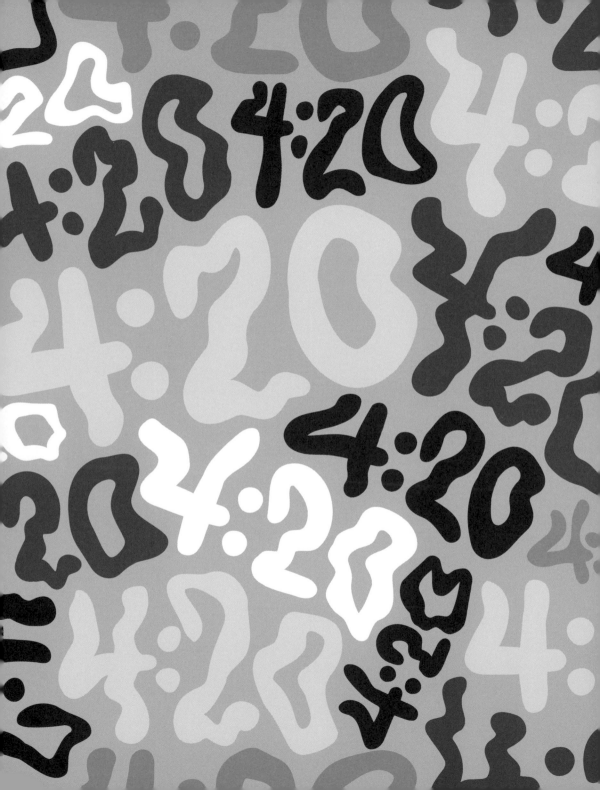

bibliography

books

Breitmaier, Eberhard. *Terpenes: Flavors, Fragrances, Pharmaca, Pheromones*. Weinheim, Germany: Wiley-VCH, 2006.

Clarke, Robert C., and Merlin, Mark D. *Cannabis: Evolution and Ethnobotany*. Berkeley, CA: University of California Press, 2013.

Danko, Danny. *Cannabis: A Beginner's Guide to Growing Marijuana*. Newburyport, MA: Hampton Roads Publishing, 2018.

Lawrence, Robyn Griggs. *Pot in Pans: A History of Eating Cannabis*. Lanham, MD: Rowman & Littlefield Publishers, 2019.

Rosenthal, Ed. *The Big Book of Buds*. 4 vols. Oakland, CA: Quick American Archives, 2001–2010.

Rosenthal, Ed. *Marijuana Grower's Handbook*. Oakland, CA: Quick American Archives, 2010.

Rosenthal, Ed, and Zeman, Greg. *Beyond Buds, Next Generation: Marijuana Concentrates and Cannabis Infusions*. Oakland, CA: Quick American Archives, 2018.

Sloman, Larry "Ratso." *Reefer Madness: A History of Marijuana*. New York, NY: St. Martin's Griffin, 1998.

journals/articles

Alger, Bradley E. "Getting High on the Endocannabinoid System." *Cerebrum* 14 (November–December 2013).

Bonn-Miller, Marcel O., Loflin, Mallory J. E., Thomas, Brian F., Marcu, Jahan P., Hyke, Travis, and Vandrey, Ryan. "Labeling Accuracy of Cannabidiol Extracts Sold Online." *Journal of the American Medical Association* 11 (November 2017):1708–1709. doi:10.1001/jama.2017.11909.

Bukinich, Dmitry D. (fl.1920-1930). "Global Plants." https://plants.jstor. org/ stable/10.5555/al.ap.person. bm000500255.

Clarke, Robert C., and Merlin, Mark D. "*Cannabis* taxonomy: The '*sativa*' versus '*indica*' debate." *HerbalEGram* 13, no. 4 (April 2016).

Cooper, Ziva D., and Hanley, Margaret. "Actions of delta- 9-tetrahydrocannabinol in cannabis." *Int Rev Psychiatry* 21, no. 2 (April 2009): 104–112. doi: 10.1080/09540260902782752.

Courtney, William. "Cannabis as a Unique Functional Food." *Treating Yourself* 24 (2010): 54.

Danko, Danny. "25 years of Chem Dog." *High Times*, September 7, 2016. https:// hightimes.com/grow/25-years-of-chem-dog/.

Fleming, Amy. "An exclusive look inside the UK's legal medical cannabis farm." *New Scientist*, July 25, 2018. https://www.newscientist.com/article/mg23931881-900-an-exclusive-look-inside-the-uks-legal-medical- cannabis-farm/.

Gardner, Fred. "Remembering Ringo." *O'Shaughnessy's Online*, April 4, 2014. https://beyondthc.com/ remembering-ringo/.

weed

Gardner, Fred. "Dennis Peron's Achievement and Ours." *O'Shaughnessy's*, December 15, 2013. https://beyondthc.com/dennis- perons-achievement-and-ours/.

Hemp Industry Daily. "CBD in the UK." https://hempindustrydaily.com/wp-content/uploads/2020/04/Report-_- CBD in-the-UK-002.pdf.

Hillig, Karl W. "A chemotaxonomic analysis of terpenoid variation in Cannabis." *Biochemical Systematics and Ecology* 32 (2004): 875–891.

Hillig, Karl W. "Genetic evidence for speciation in Cannabis (Cannabaceae)." *Genetic Resources and Crop Evolution* 52 (2005): 161–180. https://doi.org/10.1007/s10722-003-4452-y.

Jiang, Hongen, Wang, Long, Merlin, Mark D., Clarke, Robert C., Pan, Yan, Zhang, Yong, Xiao, Guoqiang, and Ding, Xiaolian. "Ancient Cannabis Burial Shroud in a Central Eurasian Cemetery." *Economic Botany* 70 (2016): 213-221. https://doi.org/10.1007/s12231-016-9351-1.

Kouliviand, Peir Hossein, Khaleghi Ghadiri, Maryam, and Gorji, Ali. "Lavender and the Nervous System." *National Center for Biotechnology Information.* doi: 10.1155/2013/681304.

Lee, Martin. "The Discovery of the Endocannabinoid System." *O'Shaughnessy's.* https://www. beyondthc.com/wp-content/ uploads/2012/07/eCBSystemLee.pdf.

Lewis-Bakker, Melissa M., Yang, Yi, Vyawahare, Rupali and Kotra, Lakshmi P. "Extractions of Medical Cannabis Cultivars and the Role of Decarboxylation in Optimal Receptor Responses." *Cannabis and Cannabinoid Research* 4 (March 2019): 183–194. doi: 10.1089/ can.2018.0067.

National Center for Complementary and Integrative Health. "Cannabis (Marijuana) and Cannabinoids: What You Need To Know." https:// www.nccih.nih.gov/health/cannabis- marijuana-and-cannabinoids-what- you-need-to-know.

Pertwee, Roger G. "Cannabinoid pharmacology: the first 66 years." National Center for Complementary and Integrative Health, *British Journal of Pharmacology* 147 (January 2006): S163–S171. doi: 10.1038/sj.bjp.0706406.

Ren, Meng, Tang, Zihua, Wu, Xinhua, Spengler, Robert, Jiang, Hongen, Yang, Yimin and Boivin, Nicole. "The origins of cannabis smoking: Chemical residue evidence from the first millennium BCE in the Pamirs." *Science Advances* 5 (12 Jun 2019). doi:10.1126/sciadv.aaw1391.

Royal Queen Seeds. "Basic Cannabis Knowledge: Genotype and Phenotype." https://www. royalqueenseeds.com/blog- basic-cannabis-knowledge-genotype-and-phenotype-n265.

Russo, Ethan. "The Case for the Entourage Effect and Conventional Breeding of Clinical Cannabis: No 'Strain,' No Gain." *Frontiers in Plant Science* 9 1969 (January 2019). doi:10.3389/ fpls.2018.01969.

Russo, Ethan. "Clinical Endocannabinoid Deficiency Reconsidered: Current Research Supports the Theory in Migraine, Fibromyalgia, Irritable Bowel, and Other Treatment- Resistant Syndromes." *Cannabis and Cannabinoid Research* 1 (January 2016): 154–165. doi:10.1089/ can.2016.0009.

Russo, Ethan. "Taming THC: potential cannabis synergy and phytocannabinoid-terpenoid entourage effects," *British Journal of Pharmacology* 163 (August 2011): 1344–1364. doi:10.1111/j.1476-5381.2011.01238.x.

Sanders, Robert. "Yeast produce low-cost, high-quality cannabinoids." UC Berkeley https://news.berkeley. edu/2019/02/27/yeast-produce-low- cost-high-quality-cannabinoids/.

Schwilke, Eugene W., Schwope, David M., Karschner, Erin L., Lowe, Ross H., Darwin, William D., Kelly, Deanna L., Goodwin, Robert S., Gorelick, David A., and Huestis, Marilyn A.. "Δ9-Tetrahydrocannabinol (THC), 11-Hydroxy-THC, and 11-Nor-9-

carboxy-THC Plasma Pharmacokinetics during and after Continuous High-Dose Oral THC." *Clinical Chemistry* 55 (December 2009): 2180–2189. doi:10.1373/clinchem.2008.122119.

Davis, U.C. "Biological Carbon Sequestration." https:// climatechange.ucdavis.edu/science/ carbon-sequestration/biological/.

acknowledgments

Society always said admitting my cannabis use would be bad for my career, but I got to write a book about it instead. Many thanks to my parents, Eric and Mary Holland, for their constant support. Thanks to my husband, Milos Cam-Robb, for always being there for me and helping me through the writing process. Thanks also to my cheerleading squad of inspiring friends, Amanda Abud, Lena Verderano Reynoso, and Megan Dooley Fisher.

The people I've met through appreciating cannabis have been some of the most brilliant, dedicated, generous and genuinely kind people I've ever met. Thanks to Eugenio Garcia for providing a creative space for flowers and talented artists to bloom on the pages of your magazine. To Gracie Malley and Todd Heath, it was an honor to make art with you for all those years. To David Downs and Ricardo Baca, thanks for believing in me and always helping to promote my work. I'll also be forever grateful to Elise McDonough for her recommendation. To my weed fairy, Angela Bacca, thank you for your constant dedication to this plant and your introductions to so many amazing people. To Ed Rosenthal and Jane Klein, it has been a blessing to become your friend. Thank you for your open hearts. For my fellow cannabis journalists and friends, especially Jimi Devine, Chris Roberts, and Mike Adams, it's always fun to collaborate with you. Thanks for shining your light my way.

This project is a love letter to a plant. Thanks to mother nature for guiding us towards living a more fulfilled life.

about the author

Ellen Holland is an Oakland, California–based journalist who has written about cannabis since 2013. Holland is the editor in chief of *High Times Magazine* and has edited several books focused on cannabis cultivation and strains.

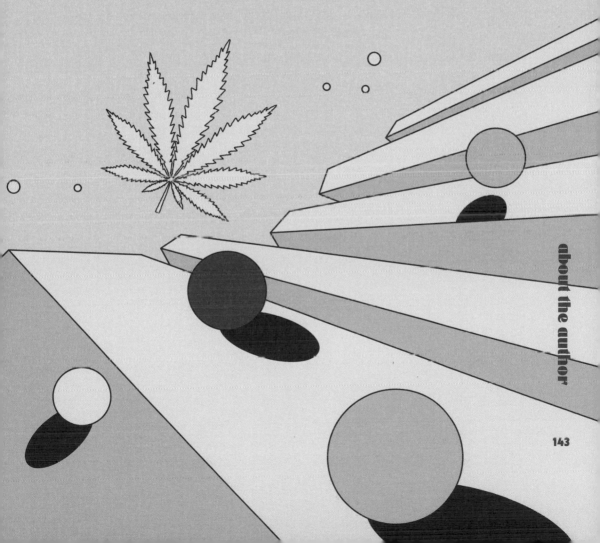

Epic Ink titles are also available at discount for retail, wholesale, promotional, and bulk purchase. For details, contact the Special Sales Manager by email at specialsales@quarto.com or by mail at The Quarto Group, Attn: Special Sales Manager, 100 Cummings Center Suite 265D, Beverly, MA 01915 USA.

10 9 8 7 6 5 4 3 2 1

ISBN: 978-0-76038-838-9

Digital edition published in 2024
eISBN: 978-0-76038-839-6

Library of Congress Control Number: 2023943240

Group Publisher: Rage Kindelsperger
Creative Director: Laura Drew
Editorial Director: Lori Burke
Managing Editor: Cara Donaldson
Editor: Katie McGuire
Cover Design: Laura Drew
Cover Illustration: Lena Besedina
Interior Design: Annie Marino

Printed in China

WEED is intended only for responsible adults of legal cannabis-use age in the United States of America, according to local state laws. Please do NOT consume cannabis and drive. If you need transportation, use a designated driver or a taxi service. And please be careful when crossing the street after consuming cannabis.

WEED does not advocate or encourage the abuse of cannabis. Please consume responsibly and in moderation. We do not, under any circumstances, accept responsibility for any damages that result to yourself or anyone else due to the consumption of cannabis or the use of this book and any materials located in it. We cannot take any responsibility for the effect cannabis may have on people. As such, we do not accept liability for any loss, damage, or inconvenience that occurs as a result of the use of this book or your reliance upon its content.